The No Bull Book on Heart Disease

The No Bull Book on Heart Disease

Real Answers to Winning Back
Your Heart and Health

JOEL OKNER, MD, & JEREMY CLORFENE, PHD

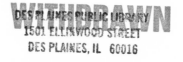
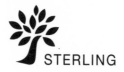

STERLING

New York / London
www.sterlingpublishing.com

STERLING and the distinctive Sterling logo are
registered trademarks of Sterling Publishing Co., Inc.

Library of Congress Cataloging-in-Publication Data Available

10 9 8 7 6 5 4 3 2 1

Published by Sterling Publishing Co., Inc.
387 Park Avenue South, New York, NY 10016
© 2009 by Joel Okner, MD, and Jeremy Clorfene, PhD
Distributed in Canada by Sterling Publishing
C/o Canadian Manda Group, 165 Dufferin Street
Toronto, Ontario, Canada M6K 3H6
Distributed in the United Kingdom by GMC Distribution Services
Castle Place, 166 High Street, Lewes, East Sussex, England BN7 1XU
Distributed in Australia by Capricorn Link (Australia) Pty. Ltd.
P.O. Box 704, Windsor, NSW 2756, Australia

Book design and layout by Scott Meola

Manufactured in the United States of America
All rights reserved

Sterling ISBN 978-1-4027-5868-3

For information about custom editions, special sales, premium and
corporate purchases, please contact Sterling Special Sales
Department at 800-805-5489 or specialsales@sterlingpublishing.com.

Dedication

To our enormously loving and supportive families: Jeremy's family: Dana, Jacob, Tess, Romy, Bruce, and Liane. Joel's family: Jodi, Sara, Noa, Mathew, Jonathon, Avi, and his mom and dad. Also, to all our patients who allow us to share in their struggles and triumphs.

Acknowledgments

It is a pleasure to acknowledge the many people who have inspired us to write this book and helped shape who we are as people and professionals. We want to thank Jeremy's three sisters Eden, Erica, and Andrea for their love and support. A special thanks to Bruce Clorfene, whose patience and editorial skills were instrumental in making our manuscript legible for our agent and publisher. We also would like to give a huge thanks to our agent Bob Diforeo and editor Jennifer Williams from Sterling whose support, guidance, and commitment continue to be a gift to their new fledgling authors. In addition, we want to give special thanks to our close friend and co-worker Sheri Marsden and her staff Trish, Tina, Joyce, Maggie, and Kim, all of whom make our jobs easier and enable us to provide the best care possible for our patients.

We would also like to thank all our inspiring instructors and teachers: Charles Merbitz, PhD, Robert Schleser, PhD, Emanuel Pollack, PhD, Christopher Comer, PhD, Ken Lofland, PhD, Rosalind Cartwright, PhD, Bruce Rybarczyk, PhD, Rosalyn Chrenka, PhD, James Wyatt, PhD, Albert Bellg, PhD, and Stuart Levin, MD.

Contents

Introduction

Why did we write *The No Bull Book on Heart Disease*? We were tired of seeing patients who were overwhelmed by and terrified of their disease not getting the guidance they needed to calm those feelings. We were tired of seeing patients who were being treated for the same problems again and again. Patients were bewildered, even lost, and had no idea how to get better. Most patients don't even know what questions to ask. Those who do ask questions don't get answers. If you are at risk of developing heart disease—or already have it—reading our book will give you a deeper understanding of what you have gone through, where you are going, and how you can get better. *The No Bull Book on Heart Disease* will not only make you feel better; it should save your life.

Performing angioplasties, lowering high cholesterol, and managing high blood pressure are simply not enough—not even close to being enough—to effectively treat heart disease. They are necessary, but unless you truly understand that your stress, six hours of sleep per night, a fifty-plus-hour workweek, a two-hour daily commute, habitual three twenty-ounce cups of coffee, forty extra pounds and poor eating habits, smoking, and a couch-potato lifestyle are the roots of heart disease, you are never going to get better.

We wrote *The No Bull Book on Heart Disease* to guide you through the heart disease process—to give you an understanding of what a heart attack is, how to deal with the hospital experience, and how to interact more effectively with your doctor, the ins and outs of diagnostic tests and medicines, and finally, an effective treatment model that you can understand and use.

We've been working together as a cardiologist and cardiac psychologist since 2001. Simply stated, our in-the-trenches tag-team approach makes our patients better. We treat each other's patients because all cardiac issues must be treated according to the individual. The resulting clinical improvements for our patients and their enthusiastic feedback form the basis of this book—a streamlined, concentrated version of what we do every day in our practice.

The *No Bull Book on Heart Disease* covers every critical cardiac topic in plain talk from the patient's point of view. We also provide equally important details your doctors won't tell you, but which are critical for heart disease victims and their families to understand if they are to successfully navigate the hitherto uncharted, frightening world of heart disease.

Let's be honest. No one chooses to have heart disease. Although there may be a strong genetic component for you—meaning that either your mother or father suffered from heart disease at an early age—it's mostly *your* lifestyle that determines if and when you are going to get heart disease and how severe it's going to be. Most people are engaged in their day-to-day existence, going about their usual business, when they develop symptoms. It can be as subtle as nagging discomfort that does not go away (chest pain, fatigue, nausea, indigestion) or it can be incredibly alarming, like feeling like an elephant is sitting on your chest. In either case, you have developed heart disease. Your heart, your life pump, is broken and needs fixing—fast! Once you have been diagnosed and treated, you enter a brand-new world with no maps or compass. It can be bewildering and frightening.

You have questions, your spouse has questions, your children have questions. Some are answered; most are not. You are told by your doctors that you can't go back to work for six weeks, you can't drive for a month, you can't lift over five pounds, and you'll be taking lots of new medicines—many of which have uncomfortable side effects—in the morning, afternoon, and evening. You are told not to have sex. You are told to quit smoking, lose thirty pounds, quit caffeine, quit drinking soda pop, stop eating red meat, cut out salt, get eight hours of sleep, eliminate stress, and take more vacations. But how do you do this? Which do you do first? What is the best approach for you?

Mentally and emotionally, you're in shock. Making so many health changes all at once is impossible. Maybe you will work on quitting smoking and trying to lower your salt intake at the same time, but addressing all the other issues simultaneously is out of the question. And you are given no guidance about how you can make the necessary lifestyle changes to turn your life and health around.

This is why we wrote *The No Bull Book on Heart Disease*—to answer all your questions about the entire heart disease process and give you both the information and encouragement you'll need to win back your heart and your health.

Here's What's in Our Book

It bears repeating heart disease cannot be successfully treated by a single health care professional. No matter how good a cardiologist may be, he or she is limited by time and expertise to provide the comprehensive care necessary to truly help most heart patients.

Heart disease patients are looking at more than just a couple of visits to a new doctor, taking a couple of new heart medicines, undergoing procedures, or surgery. The experience of being treated for heart disease is fraught with profound lifestyle changes, frightening emotions, and physical, psychological, social, and occupational changes. Successful adjustment to treatment and improved health simply cannot be achieved by seeing your cardiologist every three to six months. At a minimum, a team consisting of a cardiologist and a cardiac psychologist can begin to positively impact and change the life course of the heart patient and his or her family.

We wrote this book to describe what we do every day and to give you a simple and practical guide to how we treat heart disease. Our stories are our patients' stories, their struggles and successes. We may have our own opinions about the best way to help patients with coronary artery disease, but, in truth, our patients tell us what works and what doesn't.

Other how-to-treat heart disease books written by accomplished doctors and health-care providers don't seem to capture the essence of what cardiac patients deal with on a daily basis. Three- to six-hundred pages of *telling people what to do* has as much practical value as a build-your-own-rocket-ship instruction book. Most of these books are written with good intentions. Patients, however, need a more basic, pragmatic approach that speaks to them in a language they can understand. A glossary is provided in the back of the book to help explain medical jargon. In addition, there are dozens of sidebars throughout the text that make it easier for you to access information and tips. Sidebars with a little heart icon have been provided by Doctor Okner and address medical issues. Sidebars with brain icons, provided by Doctor Clorfone, address behavioral and psychological matters.

We believe our book provides all the important—and understandable—information that anyone who is suffering from coronary artery disease urgently needs.

Our book is divided into three parts, mirroring the chronological unfolding of the disease in three acts:

1. The initial event. In the case of heart disease, it is usually a heart attack.
2. Diagnostic tests, early treatment, and all the physical, emotional, and psychological issues that accompany any new disease.
3. Long-term, easy-to-understand and effective treatments.

The book has been written using an integrative approach that combines cardiology and cardiac psychology, which mirrors how we treat patients in our clinical practice.

PART I

Becoming a Heart Patient

What exactly is heart disease? Why is it called a disease? How do you know if you've had a heart attack? And what can you expect when you have had one? Maybe you've heard your doctor try to answer these questions using terms like coronary thrombosis, angina pectoris, and myocardial infarction— explanations that were probably as useful to you as a schematic for building a sump pump.

Part I helps you understand the basic symptoms of heart disease and what a heart attack is in terms that should go a long way toward reducing any feelings of anxiety.

1

The Story of a Heart Attack

Heart attacks do not come in "one size fits all." Heart attack victims experience a wide range of symptoms ranging from minor physical discomfort to intense, attention-grabbing pain. The story told here describes a typical heart attack similar to that experienced by many of our patients. It is told from the point of view of a male cardiac patient, although many women have similar cardiac experiences. In fact, heart disease is the number one killer of women. (See chapter 10 for a discussion of many of the unique problems women encounter when battling coronary artery disease.)

Common Symptoms of a Heart Attack

- Left-sided chest pain (sometimes the entire chest and right side are affected as well)

- Dull, aching, or toothache-like pain

- Pressure—like something big is sitting on your chest

- A squeezing sensation—like someone is squeezing your chest

- Nausea

- Vomiting

- Profuse sweating

- Dizziness

- Shortness of breath

- Pain may spread to the left arm, right arm, neck, or back

What's in a Name?

Myocardial infarction. Coronary thrombosis. Angina pectoris. Hypertrophic cardiomyopathy. Pulmonary stenosis. For you, they all add up to waking up in the middle of the night, and you don't feel right. You're sweating, short of breath, and have a pain in your chest. You get out of bed and go downstairs. You still feel bad. Maybe it's a little indigestion. You take two antacid tablets and wash them down with a glass of cold milk. You stick your head inside the refrigerator door to get some cool air and you feel a little better. You're not sure what's going on with you. Maybe it's anxiety about the big meeting you're going to the next morning. You walk upstairs and get back in bed. You toss and turn and can't get comfortable.

Now your wife wakes up because you've ruined her sleep. She asks what's bothering you. You say you just don't feel well. She looks at you and says, "You know what? You look terrible. Let's call 911." You say, "No, no, no. Just drive me to the hospital and I'll be fine."

Halfway there, you say, "You know what? I feel a lot better. Let's go back." She says, "We're going to the hospital."

In the emergency room you're nervous and don't know what to tell the triage nurse. You finally blurt out, "I'm having some chest pain." She says, "OK, we'll take you to a room and get you checked out. Can you walk twenty feet?"

Absolutely. No problem. You're a guy.

By the time you walk the twenty feet, you're drenched in sweat and the pressure in your chest is a lot worse. You take off your clothes, put on a hospital gown, and lie down. You really don't feel good.

You have now stepped out onto the floor

What to Do If You Think You're Having a Heart Attack

If you have even the remotest inclination that something is wrong with your heart, even a 1 percent chance, there are four things you should do in this order:

1. *Chew two to four aspirins immediately.* Don't swallow them whole. They're going to taste awful, but chew them anyway and then swallow. This simple step can be life-saving. It does not matter if it is baby aspirin or regular aspirin—just chew what you have.

2. *Call 911.* Yes, it's going to be embarrassing. The children, the neighbors, the dog, everyone's going to wake up, but this is a life-and-death situation.

3. *Do not convince your spouse to drive you to the hospital instead of calling 911.*

4. *Stay in bed and let the paramedics do their job.* This is not the time to start testing yourself to see what brings back the chest pain (for example, walking up and down stairs, or going outside in the cold air).

and begun "the dance." You're going to be dancing to this music for a long time with many partners. You're going to be passive and follow their lead for a lot of it.

The emergency-room doctor comes in, asks you some questions, and writes a bunch of orders. While you're wheeled out and given a barrage of tests, your wife sits in the corner of a cramped examining room holding a plastic bag with your belongings. It's clear that she feels displaced and left out.

A while later, you (now called "the patient") return to the examining room, followed by the doctor, who tells you what's going on: "Mr. Smith, we got the results of your tests. Your troponin is positive, and your CPK isoenzymes are negative. We did an EKG, and this is somewhat borderline. We're going to do some more tests, OK?"

You don't understand one word he's said, but you're too terrified to say anything, so you just shake your head yes.

Before you have a chance to calm down a little, a new team of doctors and nurses files in to take you to your cardiac catheterization (a procedure where a thin plastic tube is inserted into a leg artery in the groin area and advanced into the heart or coronary arteries. For further details regarding this procedure, please see chapter four). You're medicated and pain-free and actually feeling pretty good.

You're chatting with the team on your way to the catheterization lab, and your wife is following behind the gurney. You say good-bye to her before you disappear through the double doors.

In the lab you're lying on the table naked except for a little towel covering your groin. Lights are blaring, music is playing, and people are walking all around. The towel is whisked off, and the right side of your groin is scrubbed and shaved, and you are covered with a sterile blue drape. You're sedated and the cardiologist performs the procedure.

Next thing you know, you wake up in the recovery room. It's likely you've been slotted for one of three treatment paths:

1. Drugs, because you may have been found to have minor artery blockages and require medical therapy.
2. You may be the proud owner of a stent, a small metal tube (that looks like the spring at the end of a pen) that is inserted into a blocked artery to hold it open and allow blood to flow to the heart. It acts as a scaffolding to hold the artery open.
3. You're on your way to the operating room for coronary artery bypass grafting ("CAPG" to the medical profession; "bypass" to the man on the street).

Your old life is gone. Welcome to your new one, and get ready, you'll need a good roadmap for this one. After the procedure, you're wheeled into a hospital room. Once you are in bed, you are hooked up to an IV that's dripping into you a combination of medicines and very potent blood thinners. The doctor comes in. You've been waiting for what seems like an eternity for this guy, and now he's standing beside your bed. You're looking up at him, scared stiff. He's looking down at you, and he says, "Let me tell you what we found."

You need a decoder to figure out what he's saying. "We did an angiogram last night at about three o'clock when you came in with unstable angina. The ejection fraction is about 45 percent, which puts you borderline for heart failure. We actually found two different blockages in the mid-LAD and distal circumflex artery and put in a rapamycin-coated stent, and you should do just fine." He gives you new prescriptions, including nitroglycerin, and says, "Take this if you need it and I'll see you in two weeks. Do you have any questions?"

Do you have any questions! You've got a million of them, starting with "What the hell did you just say?" But all you can get out is "How do we arrange for the visit?"

Just as the doctor opens the door to leave, he turns and says, "OK, until I see you again I don't want any driving, no sex, no work, no lifting more than ten pounds, and no exercise. And to answer your question, the discharge nurse will help you make the follow-up appointment with me. Take care." Crazy with anxiety, you and your wife watch him go.

Once you are discharged from the hospital, until the appointment with your cardiologist, you feel at sea, set adrift with no paddles, rudder, or workable sails.

What You Cannot Do after an Angiogram

For the first forty-eight hours, you should take it easy: no running, climbing, sex, exercise, driving, or lifting weights over ten pounds. These activities won't hurt your heart, but they could cause bleeding problems at the angiogram site in your groin, which takes about two days to heal. You can assume normal activity on about day three.

Bypass Surgery

In many cases, stenting the coronary arteries, as described above, is a suitable option. But for many cardiac patients, open-heart bypass surgery is the appropriate treatment. In this case, here's how the scenario might play out.

After you awake from the catheterization, the doctor walks in with your wife. By the look on their faces you have a sneaking suspicion they've already spoken to each other and she knows what's going on. You are clueless.

Some Basic Definitions You Need to Know

Angioplasty: A procedure where a small, specialized balloon is inflated in the blocked (or partially blocked) coronary artery in order to open it up.

Stenting: After angioplasty, a very small metal scaffolding is inserted in the artery at the site of the blockage. The stent looks like and is about the same size as a spring at the end of a pen. This helps keep the artery open long-term.

Open-heart bypass surgery: A surgical procedure where your breastbone (sternum) is cut in half and new blood vessels are sewn onto (i.e., bypassing) the original blocked arteries, providing a new blood supply to the heart. The new arteries are either veins taken from your leg or arteries that supply your breastbone. They are cut out and sewn onto the blocked arteries, providing a new circulation route around the blockage.

"Well, Bob," announces the doctor, "it looks like we can't treat the blockages with stenting or angioplasty, so you're going to need bypass surgery. We'll get that set up, probably tomorrow morning."

Next, a surgical nurse comes in and gives you all the details, 99 percent of which you're never going to remember because you stopped listening when you heard the words open-heart bypass surgery.

What to Expect after Bypass Surgery

It's now a day after the surgery and you're in the intensive care unit. Here's what you should expect for the next two to seven days:

- *You will stay in intensive care for days one and two.* This is an anxiety-producing place, with machines all around you, making an incredible amount of weird noises. You hope they're good noises, but you can't be sure. The electrocardiogram machine beeps nonstop; you're worried that if it stops you're going to die, or if it beeps too fast you're going to die. Tubes are stuck into places you never imagined tubes could get into. You are totally miserable. You feel like you've been run over by a truck.
- *Days three and four are a little better.* You're out of intensive care, and most of the tubes that were in bad places (like your chest and bladder) are out, but you're still sore and not sleeping well. The trite, comic complaint is all too true—every time you fall asleep a nurse wakes you up to see if you need something.
- *On days five, six, and seven you get ready to go home.* This is good; you

feel you can do this. The nurses walk with you in the hall, working on your lungs and strength. A discharge planner works with you and everything is going really well. A discharge planner is a nurse who specializes in getting patients ready to go home.

- *Then suddenly it's time—you get to go home.* Leaving the hospital is a double-edged sword. On the one hand, you're happy to go home; on the other hand, you're a little nervous about being cut loose from the constant medical attention you've been receiving. As you leave the hospital, it's almost as if you've been reborn. You have become a "patient-citizen" living in the medical world where you're dependent on family, staff, and doctors. It's a totally different world, and you have to adjust to it.

What to Expect When You Get Home

At this point, you should be prepared to confront a number of issues:

- Your wife doesn't know how or where to touch you, and treats you like a fragile piece of crystal. This pisses you off.
- Your wife and children are scared because they've never seen you so sick and weak, and they don't know how to act. Your wife is also angry because you screwed up her life.
- You can't work for four to six weeks. Don't even think about it. And you can't drive or lift anything greater than ten pounds. You have all kinds of new medicines, new side effects that you have to figure out, and you're monster tired.
- You're undoubtedly going to be depressed. The extra stress you have now puts more pressure on any pre-existing problems you may have had such as job or family issues. If you had a problem before the heart attack, it's going to blow apart now.
- The surgical site in your leg where the catheter was inserted hurts more than your chest.

The First Post-Surgical Doctor's Appointment

Now it's time for your first doctor's office visit, and you're psyched up for it. You've been home one or two weeks, and although you're feeling a little bit better, you're still not sure about what you can and can't do. Your wife constantly

Commonly Asked Questions after Bypass Surgery

THE MOST COMMON QUESTIONS I HEAR AFTER BYPASS SURGERY:

1. When can I go back to work?
2. When can I start having sex?
3. When can I start exercising (even though the guy has never exercised before in his life)?
4. When can I drive?
5. When do I see you again?

THE QUESTIONS I *SHOULD* HEAR AFTER BYPASS SURGERY:

1. How's my heart?
2. How did the surgery go?
3. How long do I have to take these new medicines?
4. How long will it take my breastbone to heal?
5. What can I expect my life to be like in the next three to six months?
6. What can I do so I never have to experience this again?

yells at you, saying, "They must have told you five times in the hospital what your limitations are!"

The two of you walk into the doctor's office fifteen minutes early. You have fears and anxieties—and an hour's worth of questions. Your wife told you to write them down, but, of course, you didn't because you're a guy; you can remember these things. But no one ever told you that after a bypass you might have memory problems.

The doctor's office scenario is clear in your mind. You know what you want. You expect to be the first patient. The receptionist will greet you with a big smile; the nurses will embrace you and take you to a room where the doctor will answer all your questions. You're going to have a great day.

Instead, you find out there are ten people ahead of you in the cramped waiting room. You finally get a seat when somebody moves his coat off of a chair. You notice that although you have been waiting for forty-five minutes, the two people who came in after you are taken in ahead of you. All you can hear are sounds of merriment and laughter coming through the glass door that separates you from where you want to go. You're starting to sweat and your chest hurts. Or are you imagining it?

You are irritated with the other patients and office staff for complicated reasons. You hate your fellow patients because they're your competitors, even though you may never see them again. You want to get to the doctor and then get the hell out of there, and they want the same thing. Then there's the staff, the insensitive dolts who are laughing and having fun while you're sitting there in the waiting room, feeling anxious, fearful, and in pain. In your anger, all you can think about is killing the people sitting next to you and those behind the glass window.

At last the nurse calls your name. It feels like you've won the lottery because you're so excited to see the doctor after waiting an hour and a half. But do you see the doctor then? Yes, but only for a moment, as he passes you in the corridor on his way to another patient. Meanwhile, you've been led into a small examining room and are told by the nursing staff to take off your clothes and put on a supplied hospital gown. The doctor's staff then take your blood pressure, do an EKG, and ask you about all kinds of things you already answered on the form you filled out when you first came into the office.

You wait half-naked in a hospital gown for another thirty minutes, and then the doctor materializes. Here's your chance to get all your questions answered. But guess what? You've forgotten everything you wanted to ask. All of your questions about your fears and concerns are suddenly gone and . . . you're done. The doctor has hurried off to his next patient in the next examining room.

You walk out and your wife grabs you and says, "Tell me everything the doctor said!"

Some of the Most Common Fears and Anxieties Expressed after Bypass Surgery

1. I can't take care of my family. I'm going to lose my job.

2. I have lost the respect of my spouse. My family treats and looks at me differently.

3. I don't know how to get back to "normal life."

4. I am damaged goods. I am never going to get better.

5. I can't make the lifestyle changes the doctors want me to make.

6. I'm going to look damaged and ugly because of my scars.

You say, "He said I should come back in three weeks."

At this, she wants to murder you. You want to do the same to her because you know she was right about writing down your questions.

You go home and have to call the doctor and say, "You know what, I forgot to ask you some questions." The doctor does not call back immediately and you and your wife are frustrated.

2

Your Body's Warning System

Do you feel like there's an elephant sitting on your chest? Are you experiencing increased shortness of breath after sex? Does your spouse wake you and say you're snoring very loudly or that you periodically stop breathing? If you are experiencing any of these common symptoms, seek medical attention immediately. And if you hesitate because you don't want to bother your doctor, or you have too much scheduled that day, then be prepared to wipe the next two to four weeks off your important schedule while you're trying to recover in the hospital, or be prepared to meet your creator. If you are experiencing these symptoms, you must call your doctor, go to the nearest emergency room, or call 911.

People who experience a sudden onset of severe chest pain or pressure that spreads to their neck and then to their left arm should realize that they may have a heart problem and need to seek medical attention. However, most people who have heart disease don't necessarily experience these symptoms. It is all too easy to ignore and minimize the countless other physical signs that are indicators of heart disease.

Put simply, the heart is a sophisticated pump with its own electrical system. Depending upon which part of the pump or electrical system breaks down, malfunctions, or stops working altogether, you could potentially suffer a wide range of physical warnings that are not commonly interpreted as relating to the heart. Frequently, the only indication that you're having a heart problem is when you feel what are considered by most people to be non-heart-related symptoms.

Bear in mind that the symptoms described below must be considered in relation to your personal level of heart disease risk. For example, a twenty-five-year-old woman who experiences a new onset of shortness of breath while running to catch a bus is unlikely to have a heart problem. More likely she is either out of condition or has allergies. Similarly, if a fifty-five-year-old man, who has a history of high blood pressure, is short of breath as he runs to catch a bus, it is possible he has the same problem as the twenty-five-year-old woman, but he should seriously consider seeing a cardiologist.

Here are some symptoms you need to be aware of that could be related to your heart and could signal that your heart is having trouble:

- *Chest pain.* There are no *normal* chest pains. There is toothache-like pain (a gnawing, aching pain that comes and goes), pulled-muscle pain, sharp pain, dull pain, pain that is worse when you take a deep breath, pain when you're exercising, and countless others. Don't think any of these symptoms are normal. They are not. All of them need to be evaluated by a doctor.

- *Chest pressure.* It is abnormal to feel chest pressure of any type at any time, period! If you feel chest pressure when you're stressed or at rest, when you exercise, or before, during, or after meals, get it checked out.

- *Shortness of breath.* For many people, a certain level of shortness of breath is considered acceptable when taking part in any number of daily activities, such as walking up a flight of stairs. Only when it crosses a person's threshold of what they consider reasonable and normal for them does it become worrisome. Shortness of breath of any kind, however, requires medical attention.

The Real Truth about Genes and Heart Disease

Certain diseases are genetic—that is, if you have the gene you'll likely get the disease (for example, Tay-Sachs disease). Heart disease is not necessarily one of them. If someone in your immediate family has heart disease and was diagnosed with heart disease at an early age—in their twenties, thirties, forties, and maybe their fifties—you may have some bad heart genes in the family. But you need to understand that if you are in your late fifties, sixties, seventies, or older and you develop heart disease, it's hard to point a finger at "bad genes." It's a scapegoat and you are avoiding the truth about the cause of your heart disease. You need to step up and take responsibility for your disease, which is most likely due to you being overstressed, sleep deprived, over-caffeinated, underexercised, overweight, and a smoker. It is not just genetics.

- *Shortness of breath during sex.* We mention sex specifically because it is the most strenuous aerobic activity that most people engage in, and it provides an easily understood indicator of how you feel during physical activity. When you are breathing harder than usual during sex, it might indicate you have a heart problem. Most people don't get enough aerobic exercise. They often fool themselves into believing they are exercising when they walk the dog, mow the lawn, or choose the stairs instead of the elevator, when, in fact, sex is the only real aerobic exercise they are getting. Shortness of breath during sex is often one of the first alarm bells to go off.

- *Arm pain.* Our bodies are wired in such a way that you may feel arm pain if you have a heart problem. It could be arm pain with or without accompanying chest pain, and it could be either the left or the right arm. It could be pain that starts in your shoulder and spreads down to your fingers, causing a tingling sensation, or it could be a dull ache in your biceps. People often rationalize away arm pain (e.g., "I slept funny," "I strained it"). Unless you have an undeniably reasonable explanation, get it checked out.

- *Jaw and neck pain.* People who have heart disease will often report jaw and neck pain. It is usually related to exertion (i.e., exercise) or emotional stress, but not when you're chewing food. Jaw and neck pain may accompany chest and arm pain, or it may occur on its own. Either way, it needs to be evaluated.

- *Low energy and fatigue.* "I'm so tired all the time." When you feel deprived of energy for days, weeks, or months, there could be any number of reasons ranging from poor sleep, stress, bad diet, or a change in seasons, to depression, a virus, infection, thyroid problems, anemia, or heart disease. When you report low energy and fatigue during a visit to your doctor, it

Who Gets Heart Disease? Debunking the Myth

There is no one face of heart disease, although a middle-aged, overweight, slow-moving, white male smoker has been the poster boy. The bad news is that heart disease slashes across lines of gender, age, race, and social and financial status. Everybody with a Westernized lifestyle is at huge risk. Sorry, you can't feel safe just because you don't fit the stereotype.

won't necessarily lead to an immediate cardiac evaluation. However, it is a very common symptom of underlying heart disease in women and to a lesser degree in men. The bottom line is that this symptom must be seriously considered and investigated.

- *Burping or nausea.* By the time you have seen a cardiologist for complaints of stomach pain associated with meals, nausea, bloating, and excessive burping, it is likely that you have already visited your internist and gastroenterologist. It is not unreasonable to be evaluated by a gastroenterologist for these types of stomach complaints. However, you may need to see a cardiologist, as well. There are three main arteries that supply your heart with oxygen. If the front one is blocked, you tend to get arm, chest, and jaw pain and shortness of breath. If either of the other two is blocked, you don't get these symptoms; instead you may get nausea, vomiting, burping, and stomach pain.

- *Upper back pain.* The problem with diagnosing upper back pain is that everybody gets it from time to time. However, if you experience upper back pain and there is no obvious cause for it (for example, you slept funny or perhaps pulled a muscle while exercising), it could be a sign of heart disease. Before you bring this complaint to your chiropractor, personal trainer, or massage therapist, bear in mind it could easily be a heart problem.

- *Dizziness.* This is another imprecise symptom because everyone's perception of dizziness is different. Some common descriptions include the sensation that the room you are standing in is spinning around, lightheadedness after standing up, and blurred or double vision. Unless there is an obvious explanation for feeling dizzy (for example, you have a serious sinus infection, or you are on a boat or in an airplane and experiencing motion sickness), you need to be evaluated because it can be a symptom of heart disease.

- *Palpitations.* No one really pays attention to their heartbeat unless one of the following happens: you feel your heart racing for no reason, you feel your heartbeat become irregular, or you feel "stronger" extra heartbeats. Generally this feeling will not only capture your attention, but it will create a lot of anxiety. These symptoms pose a potentially serious medical issue and can easily be caused by underlying heart disease. However, unless they happen frequently, and with intensity, most people blow them off. Don't make this mistake!

If any of the above symptoms applies to you, you need a cardiologist. Don't waste any time making an appointment.

3

Eight Cardiac Patients—Meet the Faces of Heart Disease

This chapter introduces you to eight of our patients and their stories, shining a light on the human face of heart disease. Each story is unique; but together they cover a broad range of cardiac experiences.

This is how it starts: A new patient sits in our office, and we have to tell him (for simplicity's sake, we'll assume the patient is male in this instance) that he has heart disease. Naturally, he'll want to know exactly what this means. The answer to this patient's question can be answered in many ways, using any number of medical terms, because heart disease reveals itself in so many different ways. The course of the disease is dependent on who you are and the life you live. Heart disease is a lifelong illness that needs lifelong attention. It's not simply going to go away. No single definition of the disease applies to everyone. And no matter how intelligent and interested a patient may be, it is not at all unusual for him to be overwhelmed, misinformed, or uninformed about heart disease.

What follows is a broad spectrum of cardiac patients that illustrates the different nuances of coronary artery disease and what it does to real people. Each short profile outlines the basic critical factors that apply to the individual in order to give you a picture of what he or she experiences every day. Each of their lives is just as complicated as yours and can't be summed up in just a few paragraphs, but we hope the following details will give you a more tangible and personal sense of what it is like to have heart disease.

Barry

First, let's talk about Barry, 48, who lives in a suburb just north of Chicago with his wife and two teenage daughters. Barry works more than eighty hours

Barry's Key Issues

Stress. Barry works too many hours because of fear of failure.

Lack of exercise and poor nutrition. Because of the number of hours Barry works, there's "no time" to exercise or eat anything but fast food.

a week as vice president of sales for a car dealership. He has a family history of heart disease (his father and an uncle died from heart attacks in their mid-forties), an unhealthy diet, lots of stress, and no time to exercise. He is twenty-five pounds overweight.

Barry woke up one morning at about four a.m., which is normal for him because he likes to get to the office by five a.m. He felt a little funny, nothing drastic, thinking he might be getting the flu. He took a shower, after which he started to sweat, but Barry chalked this up to having the water too hot. As he was toweling off and still sweating, he remembered that on several occasions over the last two weeks he had experienced fleeting episodes of chest pressure and a feeling of warmth in his chest and left arm. He had forgotten about the episodes because they went away in two minutes.

Barry left for work at about four-thirty without waking his wife and telling her how he felt. He stopped for coffee and a muffin at a local coffee shop, and as he drove away he experienced heartburn, something he had never felt before. He got to work at around five a.m. and asked a colleague for an antacid tablet. This made him feel better, and he was no longer concerned about his physical distress.

Three hours later, Barry got up from his desk to drive to a business meeting. About halfway there, he felt a sudden pressure in his chest and began sweating profusely. The indigestion returned, first in his stomach, then traveled upward to his left breast. He said it felt like an elephant was sitting on his chest. Barry then drove to the local hospital and called 911 on the way to let them know he was arriving in a few minutes.

After arriving in the emergency room, it only took a few minutes to diagnose that Barry was having a heart attack. He could not believe this was true, because in the back of his mind Barry had always thought that if he lived past forty-five, which was the age when his dad and uncle died, he would be in the clear.

The next thing Barry knew he was lying in bed in the intensive care unit after undergoing open-heart surgery with five bypasses. His wife was crying in a corner of the room, while his daughters, who were completely freaked out, sat beside his bed. Barry didn't know what to say to them, or even where to begin.

Barbara

Meet Barbara, a lovely fifty-seven-year-old married woman with three kids. She's a control freak and a perfectionist who calls all the shots in her family. Nobody messes with Barbara. Barbara works full-time, as well as doing all the cooking and cleaning at home. To quote Barbara, "I do it all; always have and always will."

What Is the Bypass in Bypass Surgery?

During open-heart bypass surgery, new blood vessels are sewn around a patient's blocked arteries, "bypassing" the blockages. Surgeons routinely bypass between one and five blockages, but the most common open-heart surgeries involve three, four, or five bypasses. The goal is to provide a new path for blood to flow around the blockage, therefore bypassing the blocked arteries, now providing an adequate blood supply to the heart muscle.

Barbara lives in a three-story walk-up and had noticed over the last two or three weeks that she was becoming progressively more tired and short of breath when she went down to the basement with a third or fourth load of laundry. Barbara felt no chest pain, however. A week later, she went to her internist, who told her that she was probably doing too much. He suggested Barbara could be having a secondary menopause after her first one of a few years ago. He gave her no diagnostic tests and recommended a vacation in Mexico, a prospect that pleased and satisfied Barbara.

Barbara is an interesting patient. She smoked for twenty-five years and quit three years ago when her elderly father died of lung cancer. Barbara's risk factors include a history of smoking, being overweight, and being a perfectionist, which means that she is chronically stressed.

Shortly after visiting her internist, on a typical Monday morning, Barbara sat next to a woman on the train going to work. After three minutes, she knew her entire

Barbara's Key Issue

Stress. Barbara's perfectionism keeps her in a constant state of anxiety and guilt. She feels that she is the only one who can "drive the family bus"; otherwise, it will be out of control. Allowing others in her family and her life to help out or be in control is too frightening and unacceptable to her.

What Is Perfectionism?

Perfectionism describes the behavior and thought patterns of people who overorganize, overschedule, and over-control their world (including the people in their world) in an effort to cope with their own anxiety and stress. Perfectionism is often maladaptive because you can't control everything, and attempts to do so contribute to a never-ending cycle of stress.

Traditional Risk Factors

Traditional risk factors are defined as behaviors, diseases, and hereditary components that increase the chances of developing coronary artery disease (CAD). For men, these factors are a family history of CAD, high blood pressure, diabetes, overweight, smoking, physical inactivity, and stress. In the past, being a woman was not considered a risk factor for coronary artery disease because the main body of research on heart disease was done on men. For years, heart disease in women was underreported, and symptoms were ignored. In 2006, coronary artery disease was clearly shown to be the leading cause of death in women in the United States, greater than all cancers combined.

life story. Barbara's seatmate had also complained of shortness of breath, and despite multiple visits to her doctors, was never evaluated for heart problems. Within three months of her initial complaints, she had a heart attack.

The next day Barbara revisited her internist and demanded a stress test. The test results were so poor that she had an angiogram the same day, and, subsequently, a coronary artery angioplasty and the insertion of three stents.

These "traditional" risk factors apply to women, too, but for many years women's symptoms were, and in many cases still are not, taken seriously. Truthfully, this problem still exists

Bill

Bill, a fifty-year-old general contractor, is six feet tall, weighs 289 pounds, smokes, drinks, and pays no attention to his diet. His father had a heart attack at forty-five, as did his father's three brothers, all of whom were in their forties. Heart disease killed two of them.

While in Michigan's Upper Peninsula at an annual guys-only hunting outing, Bill started feeling very winded the first day out. He ignored it and followed the rest of the group. Bill was holding up OK, but on the second day he felt winded again and passed out. No one missed him because he was the last in line. Bill woke up a few minutes later and said nothing to his hunting companions because he felt better. He figured his shortness of breath and the fainting spell were the result of "nerves" and fatigue.

When Bill returned home three days later, he didn't tell his wife what happened. The following morning Bill was awakened by significant chest pressure and shortness of breath. He got out of bed and opened a bedroom window to get some fresh air. Feeling no better, he went into the bathroom and splashed water on his face. At this point, Bill threw up, which awakened his wife. She saw her husband hunched over on the sink, vomiting, sweating, and looking really pale.

Bill told his wife he wasn't feeling right and to call 911. At first Bill thought his symptoms were signs of stomach flu, which he had had before, but this time the symptoms were different and felt worse. He was taken by ambulance to the emergency room and diagnosed immediately as having a severe heart attack. An angiogram confirmed the diagnosis. If Bill had come in a few days earlier and been treated with angioplasty, he could have avoided the heart attack and more heart damage. Instead, he suffered a heart attack (his heart muscle was damaged) and then had open-heart bypass surgery two days later.

Rita

Let's look at Rita, sixty-eight, who, at only five feet tall, weighs 240 pounds. Rita smokes a pack and a half of cigarettes a day, is a type-2 diabetic, and has high cholesterol and high blood pressure. A widow of seven years, Rita has three children and six grandchildren, two of whom live with her, along with their mother. Rita was a

> ### Bill's Key Issue
>
> *Stupidity.* Bill knew he had "bad genes," but he ignored them. This is similar to a person who throws lighter fluid instead of water onto the flames that are burning down his house. Simply ignoring your genetic history does not make it go away.

> ### Traditional Risk Factors
>
> So how did we come up with these "traditional risk factors"? The initial research on heart disease was by middle-aged white men on middle-aged white male patients. Based on this research, they concluded that "traditional" risk factors are family history, high blood pressure, diabetes, being overweight, smoking, and *being a man.*
>
> These "traditional" risk factors apply to women, too, but for many years women's symptoms were, and in many cases still are, not taken seriously. Truthfully, this problem still exists.

Why Dealing Quickly with a Heart Attack Is Key to Long-Term Heart Health

Taking action as soon as possible after a heart attack is critical. Once the heart muscle is damaged, you are more prone to other cardiac problems such as arrhythmia and congestive heart failure, which result in having to take more medicines and will eventually shorten your life. Efforts to prevent a heart attack should also be a priority for everyone who is at risk.

Rita's Key Issues

Rita began her bad habits as a teenager—smoking, eating junk food, lack of exercise—and never stopped. What she is experiencing is the end result of forty years of abusing her body.

secretary for thirty years and now works at a large discount store as a stocker.

Rita thinks she knows and understands her health risks, but they don't worry her. For the last three months she has been bothered by her ankles, which swell progressively over the course of the day. When Rita takes off her shoes in the middle of the day, she finds it difficult to get them back on. When she puts her feet up after work, some of the swelling subsides, and her ankles are completely back to normal when she wakes up the next day. But for the past two weeks Rita has become short of breath when she walks the aisles of the store where she works, something she does not regard as a problem because when she leans on a cart for a minute her breathing returns to normal.

One day, Rita's daughter called her at work but couldn't understand a word Rita said because her shortness of breath caused her to speak with difficulty. Rita's daughter made an appointment with her cardiologist for the next day and had to drag her in. Rita didn't see the urgency of giving much detailed information about her condition to her cardiologist because she never thought anything was all that wrong with her. Only when her daughter provided details of Rita's symptoms did the doctor order a series of tests. Rita was diagnosed with having had a recent heart attack and congestive heart failure.

Walt

Now meet Walt, our seventy-year-old patient, who married his high-school sweetheart and has five children and six grandchildren. Walt smoked for twenty years, then stopped twenty years ago. He served in the military for fifteen years and, after leaving the service, became a tool-and-dye maker. Walt's career ended after he suffered a back injury that left him with chronic lower-back pain.

Because of the pain, Walt does not exercise. He has gained thirty to forty pounds in the last twenty years and weighs about 260, although he's only five feet eight inches tall. Walt has diabetes, high blood pressure, and high cholesterol. A couple of times a year, he sees his internist, who always tells him to lose weight and exercise more. The advice goes in one ear and out the other.

Walt's last stress test was about five years ago. He could only walk on the treadmill for three minutes because of the back pain, but was reassured by his doctor that the results were fine.

Walt was feeling sluggish, groggy, and tired, not like his old self, so he went to his doctor. Walt's wife told the doctor that he was sleeping all day. Based on how Walt was feeling and his risk factors for heart disease, his doctor ordered another stress test. Because of Walt's low back pain and physical limitation, he was given a chemical nuclear stress test, which does not require walking on a treadmill.

Walt did so poorly on the stress test that his doctor sent him immediately to the emergency room to see one of his cardiologist colleagues. An angiogram was performed that afternoon, which revealed numerous and severe blockages in all of his coronary arteries. Walt had a six-way bypass that evening.

Walt had a very prolonged and complicated post-operative stay in the hospital. In addition to having a pacemaker and a defibrillator implanted, he contracted a

What Is Congestive Heart Failure?

Congestive heart failure is a confusing medical term. Does it mean your heart is *congested*? And what does *failure* mean? Is your heart going to stop? Is death imminent? The simple answer is no, no, no, and no. Congestive heart failure means that your heart is not pumping as strongly as it should because it has been damaged. You need to think of it as a mechanical pump that is not functioning normally. Commonly, congestive heart failure can be improved with medicines and surgery.

Walt's Key Issue

In Walt's case it's all about treating what you can treat. Walt's only concern was his back pain, not his heart. Nobody ever listened to him. He had been experiencing chronic, debilitating back pain that had never been treated or addressed effectively. Clearly, he could not even attempt cardiac rehab until something was done about pain improvement.

serious infection in his breastbone. He spent ten days in intensive care and another eight days in the hospital, followed by two months in an extended care center receiving daily intravenous antibiotics and physical therapy.

Alex

Alex, a thirty-eight-year-old Hispanic cement worker, is overweight at 240 pounds. He's been married for fifteen years and has four kids. Alex was actually working at a hospital five years ago as part of a cement team building a new wing when he felt chest pain. His coworkers took him to the emergency room two hundred feet from where he was working.

Alex's Key Issues

Fortunately modern medicine saved Alex's life, but unfortunately it also failed him. Even after five stents, Alex never figured he had a problem. The procedures were so quick, painless, and easy for him that he never felt compelled to make healthy lifestyle changes.

Alex underwent an emergency angiogram and was found to have a 99 percent blockage in his main heart artery. A stent was placed at the blockage.

Alex's pain resolved immediately, and he was discharged within twenty-four hours. Over the next five years, he had three separate stenting procedures precipitated by recurring similar chest pains. At age forty-three, he had open-heart bypass surgery.

Why did Alex have severe and progressive heart disease at such an early age? Although it is true that he was overweight, Alex did not smoke, did not have diabetes, had only mildly elevated cholesterol, normal blood pressure, and no apparent stress. However, Alex does have heart disease in his family: five close relatives—two brothers, two uncles, and his dad—all died of heart attacks before the age of forty. The only reason Alex is still alive is because he had his first episode of chest pain two hundred feet from an emergency room.

Kevin's Key Issues

Kevin had a nasty combination of problems: chronic pain, major stress, sleep deprivation, and depression. There is not enough medicine in the world to control the high blood pressure of someone who has these problems. Kevin had to address his issues before he could even begin to get his blood pressure under control.

Kevin

Kevin is fifty, African-American, six feet three inches tall, and 265 pounds. He is divorced with three children and two grandchildren.

Kevin had a bad auto accident over twenty-five years ago, which left him with chronic hip and back pain. Unable to exercise, he has gained a lot of weight, resulting in high blood pressure and type-2 diabetes. Although Kevin doesn't smoke or drink, he lives on fast food.

Kevin's main issues are high blood pressure, poor diet, and enormous job-related stress. He is the regional sales manager of a pharmaceutical company where his department and product line are being phased out. It's only a matter of time before his job will be eliminated. Kevin has huge financial responsibilities, not the least of which is the fact that 40 percent of his income goes to child support and two mortgages.

Kevin has a history of coronary artery disease, and had a stent placed five years ago after a bout of chest pain that occurred at work. He did not go to a cardiologist because of his CAD, but was referred by his primary care doctor to help control his high blood pressure, which he hasn't been able to bring down, despite taking five different drugs.

Christie

Then there's Christie, thirty-eight. She's married with four children; one has attention deficit disorder (ADD), another is autistic. Christie's days are consumed with

A Review of Our Patients' Key Risk Factors for Heart Disease

SMOKING

Short-term risk: Within thirty seconds of smoking a cigarette your coronary arteries begin to constrict.

Long-term risk: Over time, smoking thickens the blood and causes coronary arteries to block up.

Constriction, clogging, and living don't go well together: Welcome to heart disease. But you can prevent this.

DIABETES

Having elevated blood sugar for years causes your coronary arteries to thicken and clog, which, again, is a recipe for heart disease.

HIGH CHOLESTEROL

Having high cholesterol for years causes fat deposits to accumulate in the coronary arteries. Progressive accumulation can cause significant narrowing of the arteries and lead to heart attacks.

HIGH BLOOD PRESSURE

The problem with years of high blood pressure is that it causes excessive wear-and-tear on the coronary arteries and increases your risk of a heart attack.

BEING OVERWEIGHT

Being overweight in itself is not the

continues on next page

problem. The problem is that overweight people have a higher incidence of high cholesterol, diabetes, and high blood pressure. This is a lethal combination for heart disease.

STRESS

The fact is, everybody is going to have stress in varying degrees. Human beings are designed to deal with intermittent stress. However, a continuously stressful life (such as one with constant marital problems, a horrible job, debt, poor sleep) will wreak havoc on your body, which in turn can lead to serious health problems including heart disease and death.

managing her children's special needs and after-school activities—doctors' visits, physical therapy, special schooling, tutoring, piano lessons, and soccer practices and games. Her nights are devoted to balancing the books of the family-owned construction business. Christie also takes care of her father, who has Parkinson's disease, and who has recently moved into their living room after the recent death of her mother.

Christie takes care of everyone but herself. She says yes to her children, her husband, her father, the business, the washer and dryer, but neglects her own needs.

She went to her doctor complaining of heartburn, fatigue, and palpitations. After evaluating her, he couldn't figure out the cause of her complaints. Only then did he refer her to our practice for further evaluation. After a stress test, echocardiogram, and routine blood tests, it became apparent that she had a low likelihood of having heart disease. However, she was at very high risk for developing heart disease in the future. Her problems were stress, stress, and more stress.

Christie's Key Issue

Christie has developed and maintained a lifestyle that perpetuates stress. She is so terrified of slowing down that she is actually speeding up. Slowing down would entail dealing with her stress.

Although the profiles of these eight cardiac patients are short, they are nonetheless emblematic of the range of the most common heart disease scenarios you are likely to experience as a patient. We are including these profiles in order that readers can get an up-front and personal view of the realities of heart disease. In chapter 22, we explain the treatment methods for each of these individual patients. The hope is that readers will be inspired to recognize themselves in these patients and discover where they lie in the spectrum of heart disease, and be invested in learning from the information detailed in the book.

PART II

What You Need to Know about Heart Disease

Has your doctor ever given you a pamphlet that explained diagnostic tests? Has he or she ever explained in plain English why you might experience chest pain or palpitations after treatment? Have the heart statistics you've read or heard from your doctor ever clarified things for you? Or do they only serve to scare you needlessly? Has the mystery of heart disease in women ever been fully explained to you? Is the role of your spouse, and the issues that concern him or her, important enough for your doctor to even mention them?

Your answer to these questions probably is: "No. They never told me that." In Part II we'll fill you in on everything you and your family need to know in order to understand heart disease.

4

Diagnostic Tests

If you are having chest pain, it is likely you will wind up in the hands of a cardiologist who will put you through a series of diagnostic tests. These tests are not designed for your comfort. Although the whole process can be unnerving, the most annoying part for most patients is waiting to be tested and then waiting some more for the results. In this chapter, we demystify and explain in simple terms what patients can expect from a wide variety of diagnostic procedures.

The Big Five

There are five main cardiac diagnostic tests: electrocardiogram, standard stress test, chemical nuclear stress test, echocardiogram, and cardiac angiogram, also known as cardiac catheterization.

Cardiac testing is not fun. Here are some of the un-fun things you will be asked to do before and during the testing:

- You may not eat for twelve hours before a test.
- You may have no caffeine for up to twenty-four hours before a test. If you regularly use caffeine, anticipate a headache from caffeine withdrawal.
- Depending on the test, you may have your groin or chest shaved.
- You may have an IV-line placed in one or more parts of your body.
- You will be lying in an uncomfortable position on an uncomfortable table.
- You will have tape applied to your body, possibly on hairy surfaces, and it may be painfully ripped off later.

Get ready for loss of control. Tests are run by technicians and nurses, and for the duration of the tests these medical workers will govern your life. They will be as nice as they can be, but they are going to tell you where to pee, what to pee into, when and where to have a bowel movement, what to lie down on, and how long you should lie down.

Insist on Being Treated Like a Human Being

Simply put, diagnostic tests can be very unpleasant, involve a large loss of control, and may make you suffer humiliation. So what do you, as a patient, want to be assured of before you undergo a procedure?

- You want to be assured that there will be little or no pain.
- You don't want to be embarrassed.
- You may be undressed or exposed during testing, and want to feel respected.
- You want a professional environment. You don't want to hear laughter or funny stories in the background.
- You want to know how and when you're going to get results of the tests. You don't want to get a phone call saying come in next week to discuss the results, and you want any explanation of the results to be devoid of technical jargon. You just want a simple call telling you that the results are OK or not OK.

Rating the Five Diagnostic Tests

In order to help our heart patients understand what to expect from cardiac diagnostic tests, we rate them according to the features that are most important to them. The description of each test covers the following points:

1. The level of pain for the patient—low, medium, high.
2. The level of humiliation for the patient—low, medium, high.
3. Specific information the test may provide.
4. Special, unique features about the test.
5. How long the test lasts.
6. The amount of anxiety the patient may experience with regard to the test—for example, running on a treadmill or being undressed in front of people, and then waiting for the test results.

Electrocardiogram (EKG)

Your clothes are off above the waist (if you are a woman, this includes your bra). The technician applies "stickies" to your chest and your arms, and wires are attached to the stickies. If you're a man, your chest will be shaved.

1. Pain level is low, but taking the stickies off and shaving the chest can be a little dicey.
2. Humiliation level is medium to high because you are undressed in front of strangers.
3. An EKG tells you how the heart is beating, as well as a lot of information about possible heart problems.
4. No special features.
5. The test lasts five to ten minutes.
6. Anxiety level is low.

Standard Stress Test

You walk or run on a treadmill for one to twenty-four minutes. Every three minutes the treadmill gets faster. The test ends when you can't walk any further, you have difficulty breathing, or you complete the test by achieving a target heart rate predetermined by your age. The entire time that you're walking or running on the treadmill you're hooked up to an EKG that's hooked up to a computer.

1. Pain level is pretty much the same as the EKG.
2. Humiliation level is potentially very high because you're exercising in front of others and you may be out of shape.
3. A standard stress test can tell you if you have any heart blockages.
4. Be prepared for a public display of sweating, shortness of breath, and body odor. No caffeine or eating before the test.
5. The test lasts from the time you arrive until you leave—about an hour.
6. Anxiety level is very, very high.

Nuclear Stress Test (Thallium or Cardiolite Stress Test)

You put on a gown and an IV is inserted in your arm. You get an isotope injection—a nondangerous chemical that is used to visualize blood flow in the heart arteries (zero harm, zero risk). Then you lie down on an X-ray table and a camera travels over you taking a picture of the blood flow through your heart arteries. You wait about twenty minutes, then run on a treadmill for as long as you can up to twenty minutes. During the last minute of the exercise, you get another isotope injection. You wait another twenty or thirty minutes and the scan is repeated. If you can't walk on a treadmill, you will be given another chemical to speed up your heart.

1. Pain level is low to high. You get an IV needle in your arm that hurts. You're lying down under a camera for twenty minutes on a hard surface and you can't move. You can have back, arm, or shoulder problems. Your arms have to be above and behind your head and cannot be moved throughout the test.
2. Humiliation level is low to high (equivalent to the standard stress test).
3. Information provided is similar to the standard stress test—it looks for artery blockages—but is much more detailed because the X-rays give a more precise diagnosis.
4. No special features.
5. The test lasts two to three hours, including an hour of waiting time.
6. Anxiety level is high due to walking and running on the treadmill and possible claustrophobia while lying still for a long period underneath the camera.

Echocardiography

You undress from the waist up and put on a gown. The technician puts lubricating gel on a probe that looks like a small ice-cream cone and presses it gently on your chest, above, around, and below your breasts.

1. Pain level is low, but sometimes the technician has to press hard if the patient is obese or has lung disease.
2. Humiliation level could be high because of being undressed and exposed to the technicians, who are strangers after all.
3. It gives a very detailed picture of how well the heart is pumping and a great picture of the heart valves.
4. You will have lots of goo on your chest that can be wiped off with a towel. Not to worry.
5. The test lasts thirty to forty minutes.

6. Anxiety level is medium, and is focused primarily on waiting for the results of the test.

Cardiac Catheterization

This is the mother of all cardiac diagnostic tests, done only in a hospital. You check in, get completely naked, and put on a gown. An IV is inserted in your arm. EKG leads are placed on your chest. Then the real fun begins. First, cold, sterile soap is slathered on the right side of your groin, which is shaved. You're wheeled to the catheterization lab, fully awake. You're transferred from your bed to a skinny "cath" table with a very hard surface. You may or may not have a pillow. Your surroundings look like an operating room—there are bright lights and cold surfaces, and the staff is busy chatting in the background. If you're given the choice, ask to be put to sleep for the duration of the procedure. There's no reason to be awake. A catheter—a long, thin tube—is inserted in an artery in your leg and pushed up into the heart arteries.

1. This is essentially a pain-free procedure with two exceptions: You will feel some mild discomfort in your groin when the catheter is being placed into the artery at the beginning of the test and again at the end of the test when the catheter is removed. You will not feel the catheter as it moves inside you.

2. Humiliation is high because you are in a hospital gown, in a cold operating room, on a hard surface having your groin exposed and worked on.

3. The test provides an exact picture of the heart arteries and tells whether or not there are blockages.

The Humiliation Factor

If you want the politically correct response to our take on "the humiliation factor," we would say that hospitals throughout the United States have a nicely framed mission statement in every room affirming their concerns about patient privacy, confidentiality, and special attention given to the human condition. But does this translate into sensitive patient care and less humiliation? The honest answer is no. The nicely framed mission statements looks great hanging on the wall, but the truth is, diagnostic testing can be humiliating. There will be times when you feel physically and emotionally vulnerable. Generally, the hospital staff do their best to provide good care and are sympathetic to most patients' sensitivities. However, be prepared to be poked, prodded, and exposed. The best thing you can do is sit back, relax, and go with the flow.

4. If you are put to sleep, the anesthetic causes an amnesiac effect that lasts for hours after the procedure. This means you have no memory of the procedure and no memory of events that occur for up to several hours after the procedure. This includes conversations with your doctor or family members. It is very common to arrive at home hours later with no recollection of what happened to you. After the catheter is removed, you will have to lie immobile for up to six hours, which could be challenging. Also, for days or weeks afterward, your leg may turn blue and have a small lump at the test site. This is normal and temporary.

5. The procedure can take from forty-five minutes to several hours.

6. Anxiety is high. The test is the most involved and technical of all the routine cardiac procedures, but the results are obtained immediately.

5 | Your Medicines

Taking medicines, while very necessary and lifesaving, can be one of your biggest nightmares. The problems are numerous, including potential negative side effects, potential negative interactions between different medicines, and confusing dosing schedules. For patients who are taking multiple medicines that result in not feeling well, it's almost impossible to figure which medication is the culprit. We have a love-hate relationship with medicines. This chapter explores that relationship and helps you understand why there are times when you just don't feel like taking your meds.

The Trouble with Meds

Medicines are not custom-made for every patient. In a perfect world, patients would take their medicines as prescribed and wouldn't suffer from any adverse side effects, but it doesn't always work that way in the real world. Here are some of the problems with taking medicines:

- It reminds you that you're sick. Each time you take a pill you look at the bottle, and think: "Man, I've got a problem."
- The cost of prescription drugs can be huge, especially if your insurance does not cover medications or you're on a fixed income.
- It reminds you that you're not in control of your life anymore. You feel like a slave to your medicines, and many people hate being dependent on anything. This fear of dependency is exemplified by the fact that you freak out when you go out of town and you forget your medicines.
- Patients are often given medicines with little education. They often are not given an adequate explanation of how the medicines should make them feel and any possible side effects.
- People don't throw out medicines that are old or have expired. This can

be dangerous. They run the risk of mistakenly taking the wrong medicine, which could be harmful.

- Patients often identify their medicines by color. We've often heard, "I take a blue pill in the morning and at night, a little white pill at lunch, and a pink pill before bed." When these patients try to get refills, it becomes challenging because health providers don't think of medicines in terms of color. To complicate matters even more, medicines, especially generics, often change color.

- Patients often do not take medications as prescribed. Why? Because you can get confused: how many, how often, when. For example, if you have five medicines of different colors, different sizes, and different doses, that should be taken at different times, it's likely you'll forget, or miss, or take the wrong amount at any given time on any given day. Weekly pillboxes can be helpful for some but useless for others who don't fill the prescription. So many of our patients have come to the office with prescriptions from their internists that were never filled because they wanted to see if they could get better on their own without taking the medicines. Patients may be sick and tired of going to their doctor with a complaint and walking out with yet another prescription, or they may not agree with the doctor's advice but don't want to tell him or her.

- They run out. In our medical system, usually a patient is given a thirty-day prescription with authorized refills. We expect our patients to take the medicine and refill it correctly. But frequently patients will take their thirty days' worth and then stop.

- Some patients experience side effects, so they stop taking their medicines.

- Some patients say they feel fine and stop taking their medication.

- A friend might tell you not to take your medicine. One of our patients ran into a cousin who said she'd heard someone on a talk show or in the pages of a tabloid say that his medicine was bad, so he stopped taking it.

- Another patient refused to take a medication because she couldn't pronounce it.

- Others simply can't remember to take their medicine, because some do affect your memory.

- Patients sometimes get confused by frequent dosage changes.

Here is an example of medicine-taking gone awry: Mr. Smith, a new patient, comes into the office. He is taking the following medications: Toporal XL 25 mg a.m. only; Lipitor 10 mg nightly; Plavix 75 mg a.m. only; Dyazide 1 mg tablet a.m. only; Altace 5.0 mg a.m. plus p.m.; aspirin 81 mg; Hytrin 1 mg tablet in the morning; Glucotrol 1 mg tablet a.m. only; Niaspan 1 tablet a.m. only; Vicodin tablet as needed not to exceed 4x/day; a multivitamin; and Viagra as needed.

When asked which medicines he's taking, Mr. Smith's answer is not an indictment of himself or of patients in general; it's an indictment of a medical system that's overloading people with pharmaceuticals. Mr. Smith says, "I'm taking a vitamin, a blood pressure pill, a water pill, a sugar pill, a pill that makes me pee more."

Can he provide any more information? we ask. Mr. Smith says, "The first one is red, the second one is blue, the third is an octagon, the fourth is oval." This is no help. He also says, "I know I'm taking Vicodin for pain." It's telling that the only drug name he remembers is the one that actually makes him feel better.

All of this leads to a basic point: If your doctor is trying to help you achieve a certain blood pressure level, glucose level, or cholesterol level, and is not successful, part of the reason may be that you are not taking the medicines as prescribed.

A big part of the problem is that our medical system is prescription-driven. As patients, we want a quick fix, and we put pressure on doctors to give us one. We want medicines for blood pressure, high cholesterol, and diabetes. We don't want to hear that these conditions can be managed to a large degree by lifestyle changes. And we don't want to hear that we have to reduce our salt intake, exercise more, eat better, and stop smoking. We want a pill and we want everything to get fixed quickly.

So this is what happens: Mr. Smith goes to his doctor's office and is told, "Look, Mr. Smith, you are overweight, you have high blood pressure, and your cholesterol is through the roof." What are the treatment options for Mr. Smith? He might be told to lose weight, eat better, start exercising, and stop smoking. Is he going to be happy with this medical advice? No! Is he going to make these lifestyle changes? We don't think so. Is he going to come back for another consultation with his doctor after having failed to change anything in six months? Probably not.

Here's a second scenario: Mr. Smith goes to his doctor's office and is given pills for his cholesterol, his blood pressure, his smoking, and his blood sugar. Lifestyle changes will be advised as an additional precaution. Will Mr. Smith be happier with scenario number two? You bet! Why? Because patients want quick fixes. They want their doctor to fix them without taking any responsibility for themselves.

As a result of this fix-fast attitude, more and more medicines are being prescribed without getting at the underlying causes of disease. But even with this fast-fix attitude people still develop a love-hate relationship with medicine because they can't cope with taking up to ten pills a day.

People understand that certain diseases require certain medicines. For example, if you are diagnosed with heart disease and undergo angioplasty and stenting, any cardiologist will prescribe aspirin, a beta-blocker, a statin, and Plavix. But unless you make the necessary lifestyle changes, you may require these medicines indefinitely.

There are two ways to look at the fact that you just had angioplasty and stenting. You can tell yourself that your life is ruined, and that you've got to take all these medicines to which you're enslaved, or you can take back control by changing your lifestyle.

Alternative Medicines

Why do patients take alternative medicines? Possibly, there are issues of control

Finding Out about Alternative Medicines

There is no single guide, pamphlet, or resource to the world of alternative medicines. Most people will seek information on the Internet. However, there are thousands of sites for every disorder, disease, and ailment under the sun—with products that claim to cure them all. There are three things you need to know to navigate this mess.

1. There are no universal standards. We don't actually know what is in most alternative products. For example, there are hundreds of brands and preparations of Ginkgo Biloba. Are they all the same? We don't know.

2. If you are taking prescription medicines, be aware that some alternative products can interfere with them.

3. Don't fall into the trap of Internet expertise. You may be an expert where your own body is concerned, but you are not an expert in alternative medical substances, no matter how much you read on the Internet. If you are going to take alternative medicines, make sure you work with someone who is an expert. It's unlikely your medical doctor will have expertise, but skilled practitioners are out there.

and trust. Patients want a say in what medicines they take, and they don't necessarily trust all the medicines doctors give them, nor should they. Above all, patients equate alternative medicines with natural medicines, and believe natural to be better. However, natural does not necessarily mean better when it comes to medications. The truth is, we just don't know.

In most cases, it does no harm if patients take natural substances or vitamins, but sometimes they interfere with prescription medications. For example, some vitamin supplements that contain Vitamin K interfere with Coumadin, a blood thinner, making it very difficult for it to do its job. Western medical practitioners of today are not trained in alternative medicine, so if you want to take alternative medicines, be smart. Make sure there are no significant interactions between the alternative medicines you are taking and the conventional drug your doctor has prescribed.

The bottom line is that the human body is a complicated, ever-changing machine. It is unlikely that the medicines you're taking today are the ones you'll be taking in six months or six years at the same dose. As your body changes, your medicine regimen must be reevaluated with your doctor on a regular basis. Eliminate the medicines you can do without and only take those you need, but always consult with your doctor first.

6

Recurrent Chest Pain

Once you become a heart patient, any chest pain you feel will seem incredibly important. You get a sudden chest pain—something you would not have given a second thought to six months earlier—and you think you are about to die. What is happening? What do you do? How do you deal with your anxiety? Read this chapter and find out.

Not Every Chest Pain Is a Heart Attack

It is extremely common for patients who have been diagnosed with heart disease, have had a heart attack, had successful angioplasty or bypass surgery, or have been treated medically for heart disease, to have recurrent chest pain. It is normal for them to focus on and be sensitive to any type of discomfort in or around their chest.

So what should you do if any of the above applies to you? The first thing is not to panic. Take a deep breath and think about the specific characteristics of the pain you are having. Is it similar to the chest pain you experienced before your heart attack, angioplasty, or bypass surgery? If that same artery clogs up again, you will experience the same pain as before. However, if another coronary artery blocks up—there are only three—you may have a different type of chest pain. If you forget everything else in this chapter, remember this:

1. A sharp chest pain that lasts from one to three seconds is not coming from your heart.
2. A sharp, shooting pain that starts in your neck and goes down your left arm to your left hand is not coming from your heart.

3. A sharp pain that worsens when you take a deep breath is not coming from your heart.
4. A constant chest pain that is with you day after day, when you are asleep or awake, during activity or inactivity, is not coming from your heart.

All of the above are likely muscular or skeletal in origin and irritating, but certainly not life threatening.

Here are the likely causes of chest pain that are not heart related:

- *Bypass surgery.* Your breastbone was split in two during bypass surgery and is now being held together with piano wire until the bone heals, which takes six to eight weeks. Every time you move your arms, take a deep breath, cough, sneeze, or even lift a saltshaker you will have chest pain.
- *Acid reflux*, also known as *heartburn.* When stomach acid climbs up your esophagus, it tends to wreak havoc in the chest area. It can cause a sharp or dull burning pain or pressure in your chest.
- *Muscle strain.* Anytime you lift something heavy, you can strain a chest muscle, which will result in some chest pain.
- *Stress.* One of the most common symptoms of chest pain is stress. If you are worried, anxious, irritable, sleep-deprived, angry, frustrated, guilt-ridden, or depressed, chest pain may not be far behind.

Chest pain in itself can cause a great deal of anxiety, which can make your chest pain even worse.

If you have had angioplasty and stenting, then you *should not* have recurrent chest pain. You might have acid reflux, muscle strain, or great stress, but your chest pain should not return. If it does, get immediate medical attention.

Finally, let's dispel the myth of the left arm once and for all: Pain that involves your left arm is not always associated with heart disease. It can be related to your neck, shoulder, wrist, muscles, or bones.

So what *do* you do when you get chest pain? While you have to be your own advocate, don't be your own doctor. If chest pain bothers you, then bother your doctor. And if you find that your doctor isn't taking you seriously and dismisses your chest pain, get a new doctor.

7

Palpitations

We've written a separate chapter on extra heartbeats, called *palpitations*, because people get them all the time, and when they do, they become very concerned. They often believe they are having a heart attack and are going to die. The fact is they are not dying, but it's important to know when palpitations should be taken seriously and how they should be treated.

Who Wants an Extra Heartbeat?

Palpitations are extra heartbeats that usually last one or two seconds. Some originate in the atrium, one of the upper chambers of the heart, others from the lower chambers, the ventricles.

Although people usually pay no attention to their heart beating, when they feel palpitations they become very frightened. Patients report a wide range of sensations when they experience palpitations:

- They may feel fluttering in their chest.
- They may sense a very strong heartbeat associated with sharp pain.
- They may experience a head rush.
- They may feel as if their heart is speeding up.
- They might feel dizzy.
- They may feel that their breath is being taken away.
- They might feel pressure in their chest.

Commonly, you may feel palpitations during a quiet time at night or at the end of the day. Palpitations commonly occur throughout the day, but you may be too busy to notice them. Most of the time palpitations are harmless, nothing more than a nuisance. But some of the time they can be a manifestation of a serious underlying heart problem.

When to Be Concerned

How do you differentiate between harmless palpitations and the ones you should investigate with your doctor? First, understand the company they keep. You need to interpret palpitations in conjunction with your cardiac risk factors. For example, if you are a sixty-year-old woman with diabetes and high blood pressure who is getting periodic palpitations, it could represent a troubling problem that should be checked out. On the other hand, if you are a twenty-nine-year-old woman with no risk factors for heart disease and have occasional palpitations, the odds are they are meaningless.

Second, consider their duration. Palpitations that are fleeting throughout the day and never last more than a few seconds are probably not significant. However, if they last for longer than a minute at a time, this should be checked out.

Third, what are the associated symptoms? If palpitations are accompanied by other symptoms such as shortness of breath, dizziness, lightheadedness, fainting, or chest pain, they should be investigated immediately.

If your palpitations begin to occur on a regular basis, or are getting more prolonged, they need to be addressed immediately. Interrupt your day and call your doctor. You can't diagnose yourself. If you are concerned, get them checked out. The more you worry about them, the worse they become. Your doctor will examine you and give you a variety of tests depending on your risk factors, your history of heart disease, and the palpitations themselves.

If the tests fail to reveal any underlying problem, you still need reassurance that you are in no trouble. You doctor should review other reasonable factors that could cause palpitations: caffeine, lack of sleep, stress, smoking, panic disorder, over-the-counter medications, marital discord, financial problems, thyroid problems, or acid reflux, to name a few.

You can see that palpitations can be, figuratively speaking, a pain in the neck. They can subject you to anxiety, a number of diagnostic tests, and possible repeated office visits.

8

High Blood Pressure

Treating high blood pressure should involve much more than just prescribing pills and then seeing the patient in three to six months. What's really needed is an individualized approach to each patient. Treating high blood pressure is not one-size-fits-all.

Is It Worth It to Take High Blood Pressure Medicine?

Most people with high blood pressure or hypertension (HTN) don't know that they have it, and that's a problem. When you're told you have hypertension and have to take medicine for the rest of your life to control it, you may feel frustrated not only because the medicine may not make you feel better; it may actually make you feel worse. Side effects from blood pressure medication may include fatigue, insomnia, and sexual dysfunction.

So is it worth taking medicine that controls your high blood pressure but makes you feel terrible? Is it worth having your blood pressure under control if the medication leaves you exhausted, sleepless, and unable to have sex? The answer is yes, with a "but." Yes you need to control your high blood pressure, because if you don't, you could have a stroke or a heart attack and die. But you should not have to give up well-being to have your blood pressure well controlled. Work with your doctor to find the right medicine that works for you and your lifestyle.

Who Is at Risk for Hypertension

High blood pressure is very democratic. It can hit anybody at any point in his or her life. It cuts across all social classes, all ethnicities, and all religions. Once you get it, it is usually with you for life.

Our patients are uniformly concerned about hypertension because they believe it causes their heart to work too hard and can lead to a heart attack. There is no question that hypertension carries an increased risk of heart attacks and heart disease. However, what is of greater concern is the risk of having a stroke, developing kidney failure, or going blind. The arteries that supply the brain, the kidneys, and the eyes are very sensitive to elevations in blood pressure. When blood pressure gets too high, arteries can leak and even rupture. This is bad.

Just What Is High Blood Pressure?

The heart pumps blood into the main arteries throughout the body. The arteries are covered with a layer of muscle that contracts and relaxes. The degree of contraction or relaxation (i.e., stiffness or looseness) of this layer determines how high or low your blood pressure is. If the arteries tighten, blood pressure goes up. If the arteries are relaxed, then blood pressure goes down.

Two numbers define your blood pressure: an upper number, called *systolic blood pressure*, and a lower number, called *diastolic blood pressure*. In general, a reasonably healthy blood pressure has an upper reading of between 120 and 140 and a lower reading of between 70 and 85. A reading of 120/80 is considered the national standard for normal.

The majority of high blood pressure sufferers were simply born with arteries that have a tendency to contract and stay contracted over time, which keeps their blood pressure elevated. Smoking, obesity, and stress also can cause arteries to contract and raise blood pressure.

Another offender is salt. Too much dietary salt results in too much water retention in your blood and in your body. When blood volume goes up, leading to more liquid inside your plumbing system, your blood pressure goes up.

As we explained, treating high blood pressure should involve much more than just prescribing a high blood pressure pill and then seeing the patient in three to six months. A comprehensive approach must be taken. An effort to find the right medicine or combination of medicines for each patient is necessary. But if you don't deal with issues such as your weight, diet, stress, smoking, lack of exercise, fifty-hour work week, two-hour commute, and sleep deprivation, just taking medicines is a waste of your time and money. You must look at the whole picture; treating with medicines alone is not enough.

The key point is that many people could get off some or at least most of their medication if they dealt with the true causes of their hypertension: smoking, obesity, poor diet, and stress.

9

Atrial Fibrillation

Atrial fibrillation (AFIB) is a condition where your heart beats irregularly constantly. This is in contrast to palpitations, which are a few extra beats now and then.

Atrial fibrillation simply means a disturbance in your heart's rhythm. Your heart is a sophisticated pump with its own electrical system. If you have AFIB, you have a short circuit in your wiring system that causes your heart to beat irregularly.

These are the common causes of atrial fibrillation:

1. *Long-standing high blood pressure.* Chronic high blood pressure wears out the heart muscle, which can lead to AFIB.

2. *Coronary artery disease.* Blockages in heart arteries often damage the heart and lead to AFIB.

3. *Rheumatic heart disease.* Rheumatic fever is a childhood illness, uncommon in the United States today. Having contracted rheumatic fever as a child can lead to heart valve problems with AFIB as an adult.

4. *Thyroid disease.* Think of your thyroid gland as your internal battery that regulates your metabolism. If it is either over- or under-active, it can cause AFIB.

5. *Pulmonary embolism.* A disease where blood clots form in your lungs, often due to prolonged sedentary behavior, such as long hospital stays, or long airplane or car rides.

6. *Chronic alcohol use and abuse.* Alcohol is a heart poison, and one of the toxic effects of alcohol is AFIB.

7. *Just plain bad luck.*

Treatment Strategies

If you develop atrial fibrillation, you either feel it or you don't. Patients generally fall into two broad groups. About 40 percent don't feel anything; in fact, they don't even know they've developed AFIB. The other 60 percent plain feel bad. They feel as though their battery has run down. They're tired, short of breath, have difficulty exercising, and just have a hard time getting through the day. They feel like they have gotten very old very quickly.

There are three different aspects to the treatment of atrial fibrillation:

1. *Rate control* is a treatment strategy in which patients are given medicines just to slow down the irregular heart rate, not to eliminate AFIB. The symptoms of AFIB are eliminated in patients who respond to the control.

2. *Rhythm control* completely eliminates AFIB by restoring normal heart rhythm. This is done either with specific medicines called *antiarrhythmics* or a procedure called *electrical cardioversion.* You are born with normal rhythm, which is termed *normal sinus rhythm.* Many patients feel better when they are back in normal rhythm.

   Thus, the goal of rate control is to eliminate the symptoms while leaving the patient in AFIB. The goal of rhythm control is to eliminate AFIB completely. However AFIB makes you feel, another significant problem is the risk of a stroke. Put simply, blood clots can form in the heart when it beats irregularly; these clots can travel to the brain and cause a stroke.

3. *Anticoagulation,* the third strategy of AFIB treatment, requires the use of blood thinners. If AFIB is treated with a rate control strategy, blood thinners are required. If a rhythm control strategy is used, blood thinners are not required because the AFIB is eliminated and the risk of stroke is eliminated as well.

The Problem with Alcohol

When ingested, alcohol is a poison. Whether it's rubbing alcohol, wine, beer, or bourbon, choose your poison. It affects your brain, nervous system, liver, stomach, kidneys, and pancreas, to name a few. Although this is common knowledge, most people don't know that alcohol is also a serious heart poison. The more and longer you drink, the more it affects and damages the heart muscle. Congestive heart failure can occur if you drink excess alcohol over a prolonged period of time.

So, wouldn't it be better to try to put all patients back in normal sinus rhythm? The answer is probably yes, but this result is not always obtainable and has to be approached case by case.

Blood Thinners

The medicine most commonly prescribed to minimize the risk of a stroke in patients with AFIB is a blood thinner called Coumadin, or warfarin, with aspirin considered a second choice. Blood-thinner drugs, while often necessary, have specific side effects and limitations, which most patients find very unpleasant. These are some common issues with Coumadin:

- Bleeding and bruising. A small cut from shaving can result in significant bleeding, and even bumping into something gently can cause unsightly bruising underneath the skin.
- Need for frequent blood tests at your doctor's office to check how thin your blood is.
- Monitoring everything you eat at every meal and snack because different foods can either cause Coumadin to become ineffective and put you at higher risk for stroke or increase its effectiveness, which can heighten your risk of bleeding.
- Being tied to medical therapy indefinitely.
- As long as you have AFIB, you require anticoagulation, which means spending more time in your doctor's office.
- While Coumadin significantly decreases the risk of stroke, it does not eliminate it completely. In many patients aspirin does

What about Red Wine?

There are buckets of research indicating that moderate *red* wine consumption (four to six ounces per day) may have some heart benefits. The truth is there are way too many confounding lifestyle factors such as amount of exercise, type of diet, smoking, stress, and strong family history that influence your health and heart more than a glass of wine. The real problem is that it is ridiculous to think that someone who is overweight, eats poorly, does not exercise, and smokes is really protecting his or her heart with four to six ounces of wine per day. Recommending moderate wine consumption on the basis of this research is equally absurd. Sorry, wine lovers. In addition, we are not confident that most people will actually limit their consumption to one four-ounce glass. We realize that alcohol is a pillar of our culture and is often used as an anesthetic to take the edge off a hard workday, but we cannot recommend it as a heart-healthy strategy.

as good a job as Coumadin without the unpleasant side effects, a fact that needs to be determined by your doctor.

Food Interactions with Coumadin

Almost every patient on Coumadin has a strong desire to get off of it because it's a major pain in the neck. All foods that contain high levels of vitamin K—including anything green and leafy, such as lettuce, spinach, kale, collard greens, Brussels sprouts, scallions, turnip greens, and even green tea—counteract the effects of Coumadin.

Because there are so many foods that negatively interact with Coumadin, it's necessary to measure Coumadin blood levels on a regular basis, usually monthly but sometimes as frequently as every week. Patients hate this because they're tied to medical therapy, have to worry about what they eat, and are constantly concerned about where they're going to go to get their next blood test.

The Bottom Line on Atrial Fibrillation and Coumadin

1. Try to find out the cause of your AFIB—alcohol, thyroid disease, heart disease—because if you can find and eliminate it, you may be able to eliminate the AFIB and everything that goes with it.

What Is Electrical Cardioversion?

Electrical cardioversion is a less-than-one-second procedure that takes place in the hospital (while you are sedated) that shocks your heart back into normal rhythm. As scary as it may sound, there is no pain involved, and patients awaken thirty minutes later with no memory of the event.

Warning!

If you are taking Coumadin, you are trying to thin your blood. Any green, leafy foods or beverages that contain high levels of vitamin K are going to prevent Coumadin from working. Sorry to all you broccoli fans and green tea lovers out there: Don't eat or drink this stuff while on Coumadin.

Coumadin vs. Aspirin

According to the American College of Cardiology, the sicker you are (as a result of diabetes, history of stroke, history of heart attack, congestive heart failure, high blood pressure, or advanced age), the better your chances of not having a stroke if you take Coumadin as compared with aspirin. Conversely, an otherwise healthy young person with AFIB would do just as well with aspirin instead of Coumadin.

2. Work hard to find the treatment that works for you, either rate control or rhythm control. Don't compromise your quality of life; you have to feel good while taking the medicine. Discuss this with your doctor, because these days treatments can be adjusted to find the right mix for you.

3. Anticoagulation, through the use of a blood thinner, is a huge problem for most people. Work with your doctor to get off this medicine if it is at all possible.

10

Women and Heart Disease

Most health care professionals do not listen well enough to women patients, nor do they take them as seriously as male patients. We strongly believe this is the major reason why heart disease is the number one killer of women in the United States. This chapter pulls no punches in explaining why women's heart disease is underdiagnosed.

Misinterpreting Women's Symptoms

According to the American College of Cardiology, more women die of heart disease than of breast cancer, lung cancer, ovarian cancer, respiratory diseases, and diabetes combined. We strongly believe there are two major, but not commonly discussed, reasons for why this is true of women of all ages:

1. Women patients are not listened to, and are not taken as seriously as male patients, by doctors.
2. There is a large subgroup of women who have heart disease but don't show classic cardiac symptoms.

When a woman finally gets her ten-minute meeting with a doctor, she is fighting an uphill battle from the beginning. We believe there is an inherent bias against women by both male and female doctors with regard to interpreting their expressed symptoms. Men are less likely to communicate how they feel physically or express what their emotions are when they're not feeling well. Therefore, when they finally do talk about themselves in these terms, their symptoms are more apt to be taken seriously by their physicians because they must be "real." Women's symptoms, on the other hand, are often seen merely as "complaints" and are not taken seriously.

If you look at men and women whose risk profiles for heart disease—age, hypertension, high cholesterol, diabetes, smoking, family history of heart disease, stress—are demographically similar, men receive more diagnostic testing than women who report similar complaints to their doctor.

When a fifty-year-old man walks into his doctor's office complaining of chest pain, he will immediately receive a full complement of cardiac diagnostic tests. A fifty-year-old woman expressing the same complaint may be given the same barrage of tests, but very likely only after other medical problems have been considered as the cause of her chest pain, such as anxiety disorders, stomach problems, menstrual issues, thyroid problems, and so on.

Here's the root of the problem: Women's reported physical symptoms are often not recognized as cardiac in origin. The number-one complaint that will alarm any doctor that their patient has a heart problem is chest pain. The problem is that while women often report chest pain, they describe it differently than "classic chest pain," which is defined as pain or pressure sensation on the left side of the chest, which may or may not spread to the left arm or left side of the neck. Women's chest pain can vary in occurrence. It may be right-sided, an upper back or upper abdominal pain, a fleeting chest pain associated with fatigue or shortness of breath, or the pain may be diffuse or nonspecific. These chest pains that differ from the classic chest pain more often reported by men are called *atypical*. This misnomer is critical because in the medical culture *atypical* anything is often considered less important and can result in less aggressive diagnostic testing.

Classic vs. Atypical Chest Pain

Women's chest pain is not *atypical*—in fact, it is *typical* for women. Why is there an expectation that men and women should experience chest pain the same way? Although men and women may differ by only a single chromosome, their physiology is different and may manifest different symptoms. If medical practitioners call a woman's chest pain "atypical," it is because male doctors have written the textbooks and are the ones who define chest pain. If a woman's symptoms don't fit any of their definitions, her pains are considered atypical. This is not only a ridiculous state of affairs, but it is also a very grave problem for women. It bears repeating that at the end of the day doctors run the risk of minimizing or negating women's chest pain or other symptoms because they have been trained to call it "atypical" and take it less seriously than classic chest pain. Again, they identify men's chest pain as real, implying that women's chest pain is less real, less severe, and warrants a less thorough investigation. Rarely does a man receive a diagnosis of atypical chest pain.

We believe a more meaningful approach to understanding, diagnosing, and treating a woman's symptoms is to classify them according to her pre- or postmenopausal status. Current medical thinking holds that women's hormones may have a protective role and play a part in guarding against heart disease. We say "play a part" because women's hormones may not *necessarily* protect women, but rather affect how heart disease makes itself known. Postmenopausal (older) women with heart-related symptoms are more easily diagnosed, while premenopausal (younger) women with heart disease are underdiagnosed. Discussing women and heart disease in terms of hormonal status allows us to remain consistent with some contemporary practices and enables us to make some critical observations that will help women better understand how to describe their symptoms to their doctors. In order to do this, we broadly define two diagnostic groups: postmenopausal women and pre- and perimenopausal women (before and during menopause).

Men tend to have their first heart problems diagnosed when they are in their fifties. Women are more apt to receive the same diagnosis in their sixties and seventies. The only explanation for this is that postmenopausal women most often describe their heart disease symptoms—chest pain, arm pain, neck pain, chest pressure, shortness of breath with exertion, such as walking up stairs—in the terms that men use. Since these complaints are similar to the typical coronary artery disease symptoms described by men, doctors diagnose heart disease in these women much more readily.

Women in their sixties, usually postmenopausal, get the same frequency of diagnostic heart testing (stress test and angiograms) as men of the same age, while women in their thirties, forties, and fifties receive less heart testing than men in the same age group. Consequently, pre- and perimenopausal women with heart disease are in big trouble, because they tend to present their doctors with a wide array of symptoms that don't seem to be related to the heart but in fact are. This is where doctors run the risk of underdiagnosing. Please note that it's possible for some younger women to describe typical symptoms such as chest pain and pressure, but it's not common.

Pre- and perimenopausal women often report symptoms that are not commonly interpreted as indicative of underlying heart disease because doctors and patients alike "know" that younger women have lower incidence of coronary heart disease. This makes it more likely that the doctor can miss the diagnosis. This means that when a premenopausal woman visits her doctor with complaints atypical of heart disease, the doctor will likely shuttle her to a cadre of specialists looking for non-cardiac causes of her problems. She will get stomach and bowel tests, thyroid tests, chest X-rays, blood work, and possibly be given a prescription for antidepressants or antianxiety medicine. Often, it is only when these tests and treatments don't help that heart tests are considered.

A Fresh Approach for Women and Heart Disease

We say it is high time for a broader, sounder approach to women's cardiac symptoms. It is a fact that premenopausal women do contract heart disease, and with the current trend of increased obesity, high cholesterol, diabetes, and stress, doctors must make heart disease an initial consideration.

Doctors *and* women need to understand that coronary artery disease is a real issue for both pre- and postmenopausal women. A woman's "atypical chest pain" and other nonclassic cardiac symptoms should be initially investigated with heart disease in mind as a potential primary cause. The results of a stress test will determine what additional diagnostic or treatment options are needed.

Michelle's Case

Michelle is forty-four, married, and the mother of three children. She smokes and is mildly overweight. Michelle has a family history of heart disease—both parents had heart attacks in their late sixties and early seventies. She works part-time in an accounting office and enjoys her job. Michelle felt "sluggish" for weeks, which she thought was either due to a cold or the flu, and was not sleeping well. She also felt shortness of breath and sporadic chest discomfort for the past two months.

Michelle finally visited her internist, who evaluated her and performed blood tests, which came out fine. He concluded that because it was income tax season, she had been working longer hours and the stress was taking its toll. He prescribed two weeks of sleeping pills, recommended she quit smoking, and told her to cut back her working hours.

Within two weeks, Michelle returned to her doctor with no improvement. He then prescribed a strong antacid and antireflux medicine to address her chest discomfort. Again, there was no improvement. Michelle also noticed that her shortness of breath was getting worse, which she attributed to poor sleep and continued smoking. When she told her mother she wasn't feeling well, her mother told Michelle to call her own cardiologist. Michelle thought her mother was being an alarmist, but to get her off her back she agreed to see him.

 Men's and Women's Symptoms

Men: Chest pain, chest pressure, arm pain, jaw pain, nausea, sweating, shortness of breath.

Women: Chest pain, chest pressure, arm pain, jaw pain, nausea, sweating, shortness of breath, sharp chest pain, right-sided chest pain, fatigue, upper back pain, upper abdominal pain, a fleeting chest pain associated with fatigue or shortness of breath.

After meeting with Michelle, the cardiologist told her, "It is probably nothing," but set her up with a stress test later that week. She did poorly and was sent to the hospital for further cardiac testing—a cardiac angiogram. It showed she had one coronary artery that was over 99 percent blocked, and a second artery 90 percent blocked, and that in all likelihood she was on her way to a massive heart attack. Michelle underwent angioplasty and stenting, which effectively opened up her coronary blockages. Soon after the procedure, her symptoms disappeared. Michelle was committed to serious lifestyle changes because she was fed up with feeling tired (this was her "hook"; see chapter 16).

This story is all too typical. It is critical for woman of all ages to consider cardiovascular disease as a possible cause when symptoms (e.g., fatigue, shortness of breath, sporadic chest discomfort, nausea) show up. We hope they are due to other, less serious causes, but too many women suffer irreversible harm because a diagnosis of heart disease was simply not considered.

11

Treating the Untreated Patient

With the diagnosis of heart disease, typically first indicated by a heart attack, the medical focus should be on the patient. But what about the needs of his partner? In an instant, both of their worlds are turned upside down, the level of their dependency on each other is suddenly reversed, and the dynamics of their relationship are put to the test. Under these circumstances, the spouse simply cannot be ignored—as she most often is. (In this chapter, we're going to use the wife as the spouse of the cardiac patient, although as the population ages the roles are often reversed.) In fact, her medical, psychological, and social needs must be integrated into her husband's treatment plan, since his well-being, when all is said and done, is largely dependent on his partner's well-being. This chapter is dedicated to her.

Taking Care of the Spouse

Although the focus should be on the patient from the time he is diagnosed with cardiovascular disease, it is his spouse who often takes the bigger hit. She can easily be in shock, feel overlooked, and be overstressed. But nobody is dealing with her issues.

Think about it. He wakes you up in the middle of the night and says, "Honey, call 911; I think I'm having a heart attack." All you can think about is whether he's going to die. You call the paramedics, who arrive and race to your husband, who is hunched over on the edge of the bed. All their attention is on him.

Your problems begin *now*, as you become a spectator to the events unfolding before you, and over which you have no control. Your needs, questions, and issues are ignored, and it will get much worse. The focus of events shifts from your house, to the ambulance, and then to the hospital emergency room.

Your husband is now officially sick—a patient lying on a bed wearing a hospital gown. He's having intense chest pain and feeling very uncomfortable. Nurses are coming in and out of the room taking blood samples, doing an electrocardiogram and a chest X-ray, waiting for the doctor to arrive.

Where's the patient's wife? You're sitting on a stool in a corner with a pile of coats stacked on your lap, holding your husband's belongings in a plastic bag, being completely ignored. You feel a wide range of emotions—the prevalent ones being anger and fear. What's happening will disrupt your entire life.

The doctor arrives and reviews the results of the tests. He tells the patient it looks like he's having a heart attack and needs an emergency angiogram. Your husband is whisked away to the cardiac catheterization lab. You walk behind him, but as he goes through the double doors bearing the sign "Do Not Enter," you get sent to a waiting room. It's the middle of the night, you're sitting by yourself, and no one's telling you anything.

What happens next? The patient undergoes a cardiac angiogram that can lead to three possible treatment paths: medications, angioplasty and stenting, or open-heart bypass surgery. In this case, the patient will undergo open-heart surgery, and we will tell the story of this procedure from the spouse's standpoint.

How It All Looks from the Spouse's Point of View

The patient—your husband—is now put through an invasive, three- to six-hour operation. What about you? There you sit in the surgery waiting room knowing little or nothing about what your husband is going through. Sometimes the surgical nursing staff takes you on a tour of the intensive care unit to see what other patients look like after surgery, and then follow up the tour with a ten-minute teaching video about open-heart surgery. This only intensifies your fears and loss of control.

The part of the video you're likely to remember is the place where it shows the patient's heart being stopped for approximately thirty to forty minutes during the operation, a necessary part of bypass surgery. This creates even more stress, as you interpret this as "My husband will actually be dead for half an hour," followed by the inevitable question: "Will they be able to restart his heart?" You then wait anxiously for someone from the surgical team to come out and give you a progress report on the surgery. Unfortunately, you often have to wait until the six-hour operation is over to get any meaningful news.

Thirty Minutes Without a Heartbeat

Surgeons can't operate on a moving target, so they need to stop the heart for part of the bypass operation. During this time, the heart-lung machine takes over the breathing and pumping responsibilities for the body and the surgeon is able to sew the bypasses in place. The heart is restarted about thirty minutes later.

When hours pass with no word, you begin to think: "My God, they couldn't start his heart again." You're so overwhelmed you can hardly breathe. All you want is to know that your husband is fine. You don't care about any of the technical aspects of the surgery, although you will later.

At this point, the intensity of the waiting room must be described. Typically, there are a number of families waiting to hear about the results of a loved one's serious operation. It becomes intensely competitive each time the operating-room doors swing open and a doctor walks through and searches for a member of his patient's family. You want the doctor to be yours, with the information about your husband. You don't care about anyone else's. Your stomach is doing flip-flops in anticipation.

How's My Husband?

When your doctor finally emerges, he spots you and begins his report. You just want an answer to "Is he going to be OK?" Reflecting on his handiwork, the surgeon will give a somewhat technical description of the operation. When he leaves, after giving you positive news, you can now digest the information. The problem is there is very little to digest. All you heard was "Blah, blah, blah . . . artery, bypass, pump . . . He is resting and doing OK. You can see him in an hour."

You now have to make the necessary phone calls to everybody waiting to hear what happened. The problem is you did not hear any of the details and you are in a state of anxiety until you can track someone down who can provide descriptive and pertinent medical information about the operation that you can understand.

After the surgery, it normally takes about an hour to transfer a patient to the intensive care unit (ICU) and settle him in. You and other family members are invited in. It is here where your worry and anxiety are highest. You are terrified to see what your husband is going to look like. You find him sedated, intubated (with a breathing tube in his mouth), and with more tubes going in and out of his body than can be imagined.

You are too overwhelmed at the sight to focus on your husband. Rather, as the hours go by, it is the sound of all the machines that are keeping him alive that grab your attention: the beeping of the EKG machine, the suction coming from his chest tube, the breathing sound of the respirator, and the constant humming of the intravenous pump. You're listening to the idle chatter of the nurses at their station, which only heightens your anxiety because all you're thinking is "why aren't they in here watching my husband?" Invariably, the first question you'll want to ask is "Can I touch him?"

When you do take a good look at your husband, who you're sure is barely alive, you're thinking, "This is not what I signed up for." This is a defining moment for you as you reprocess every aspect of your life together, past, present, and future.

Navigating "Post-Op"

During the next twenty-four to thirty-six hours the patient wakes up, the breathing tube comes out, and one by one the other tubes are removed as well.

He feels as if he's been run over by a train. Every part of his body hurts. Every bodily function causes pain—hiccups, breathing, urinating, coughing, trying to sit up—all making him very difficult to deal with.

As a rule, post-surgical heart patients spend the next three to five days in the hospital and then are sent home. As his spouse, what do you have to deal with now? You have a guy who has had bypass surgery who tells you he just wants to get stronger so he can go back to work. He's not interested in being lectured; he does not want to hear that he can't do this or can't do that.

His main concern is to feel better. He's still feeling all sorts of pain: chest pain

A Key to Surviving Your Spouse's Surgery

Surviving your husband's surgery is about acceptance. For the most part, you will be overwhelmed, underinformed, and frustrated. You are an outsider looking in. The orderly pushing the gurney has more insight into the hospital routine and your spouse's surgery than you ever will. Grab any and all information you can to help you get through it, but understand that you have little to no control over what is happening, and have to simply accept this fact.

Support Options for the Spouse during and after Heart Surgery

The fact is you are not the prime focus of the doctors or other hospital staff. You are overlooked more often than not. However, services are available to help you with information and support. But you have to ask for them. Here are some options:

- A *chaplain* is available twenty-four hours a day and is a good source of support and information about what to expect next.

- *Hospital patient representatives* are also usually available during daytime hours to provide support and information.

- *Heart Menders* belong to an organization only for people who have had bypass surgery or their spouses. They can be contacted before or after surgery to offer insight and support.

because they cracked open his breastbone; leg pain from where they took veins for his heart and an inability to bend the leg because it's so stiff.

He can't sleep and can't roll over on his side because he can feel his breastbone move when he does. This really unnerves him. When he tries to open a door he feels more pain because the breastbone keeps moving.

He has significant limitations for the next four to six weeks. For example, he is not allowed to lift more than five to ten pounds, drive a car, or go back to work for at least a month. And the last thing he wants is to discuss lifestyle changes with his spouse.

You, on the other hand, only want to tell him in no uncertain terms: "You are not going back to your old ways. The reason our life has been turned upside down is because you screwed up and let this happen to you. We're not doing it your way again."

His response? "We'll talk about it later."

When you hear this, you feel a huge surge of stress. You're angry, frustrated, scared, and depressed, all at once. This is a very difficult and challenging time for you. Patience with him is either gone or reduced to almost nothing, particularly when he wants to go back to his "bad" habits. You would like to kill him.

Although you and your husband have begun a new life, he is going to get direction and guidance. You're going to get nothing. Your needs are going to be pretty much ignored by the doctor. The focus will be on the patient, and in some respects it should be. But you're the patient's spouse, and you have to pick up where he left off. There are bills to be paid, there are kids to be raised, the family has to be fed. There are a multitude of obligations, and you know what? All of a sudden you have to meet all of them. If you didn't have stress before, you're surely going to get it now.

Welcome to Your New Life

Hopefully, your family will provide you with some support after your husband's surgery. But more often than not, you're on your own. This is your life now, and it's presenting you with a host of challenging issues.

- *Changes in responsibilities.* Your life was neatly delineated before the heart attack—your husband had his role, you had yours. Now your routine, your boundaries, your guidelines are all up for grabs. You're the wife of a once high-functioning guy, and as such, you had a certain role with certain responsibilities, but now that's all gone. You are now a caretaker, and you could easily be the family's sole provider. And you don't necessarily want the new job.

- *Sex.* Most of what your husband is going to think about after he starts to feel better is how soon he can have sex. Are you even thinking about sex? It has disappeared from your mind. This guy is a cracked egg who might break if you just touch him. You're thinking: What is wrong with this guy? How can he think about sex when our world has been turned upside down?

- *Anger.* "I told you this was going to happen. It shouldn't have, but it did because you went and had two helpings of baby back ribs with extra sauce and fries. I told you to go to the gym and exercise. I told you to stop smoking. I told you we needed a vacation, and you said 'I don't have time.'"

- *Fear.* You're freaked out of your mind with fear. Is he going to die? Is he going to be permanently disabled? Is he going to lose his job? Do we have enough money to pay bills? Is this going to affect whether or not our kids go to college? We were going to retire at age sixty-five, and now he's sixty with $160,000 in hospital and doctor bills. Do we have to sell the house? Do we forget our plans and dreams?

- *The porcelain doll effect.* You may look at the patient—your husband!—

as fragile and weak. Consequently, your worries keep you up at night. Your doctor gives you sleeping pills and takes the time to ask you why you're not sleeping. You tell him you're up nights watching to see if your husband's going to stop breathing. You say, "I put my head on his chest, and he thinks I'm cuddling and he starts thinking about sex. But no, I just want to make sure his heart is not going to stop. I just need reassurance that my husband is not going to die."

- *The patient himself.* In the first month home, he's doing a whole lot of nothing. He can't lift more than ten pounds, which happens to be the average weight of a full bag of groceries. He's afraid to do anything, so he tends to do nothing. He's frustrated and bored. All you and he do is look at each other. He watches TV and you watch him.

Rejoining the World

A month has now passed since your husband's heart surgery. What changes have occurred? He can return to work on a part-time basis. He can drive. He will likely begin a cardiac rehabilitation program, such as a supervised exercise program meeting three days a week for one hour a day with additional education and psychosocial evaluation (see chapter 18). The restrictions are easing, and life is getting back to a more normal routine.

Theoretically, you and your husband can begin to have sex again, but there are some issues that often get in the way:

- If you weren't that interested in sex before the surgery, you certainly don't want to have it now. Your husband may be concerned about his ability to perform and asks about Viagra. You tell the doctor, "If you give him Viagra, this is the last time I'm bringing him to your office."

Myths and Realities about Sex After Surgery

Having sex after bypass surgery will not cause a heart attack. In fact, you could actually have sex as soon as you are transferred out of the intensive care unit. You have a new blood supply to your heart.

But you do need to heal first before having sex. The combination of your breastbone being held together with piano wire, several leg wounds where veins were removed for bypass, and the recent removal of your urinary catheter make having sex more than a little uncomfortable and challenging. It is better to wait a little while.

- You also have no interest in sex because you think it might injure your husband or risk the possibility of another heart attack.
- Your husband may not be interested in sex because he is frightened that it could give him another heart attack. He also struggles to achieve an erection because of this fear, and because he may be on medications that have sexual side effects. Consequently, he avoids sex altogether rather than risk being humiliated.

Health Police

You now have the responsibility for defining everything your husband has to do. You tell him to eat better, cut out the salt, stop smoking, cut back on drinking, take his medicines, and start exercising every day. You are much more open to making positive lifestyle changes. You want to go in a new direction, especially with diet and exercise. You even offer to go for evening walks with him so he can get his daily exercise. All he's thinking is "I'm going to get though this. I'm going to be fine, and in six months I'll be back doing what I want to do."

How to Deal with Anger

Anger is an outward expression of inner pain and frustration. Your anger is probably completely justified. However, remaining stuck in an angry state does not allow you the freedom, creativity, and insight to address any of your life's problems. So, you need to cool down and decompress from this state in order to truly deal with your issues. Some helpful strategies are to go for a walk, walk the dog, do yoga, ride a bike, play basketball, lift weights, call a friend and vent, take a break from the kids, take a shower or bath, or try deep breathing. Usually *any* physical activity helps burn off some anger. Also, putting some distance between you and what's making you angry helps. However, eating sweets and junk food, smoking, drinking alcohol, or yelling will truly only make the situation worse. Whatever it takes to cool you down before dealing with an issue is key.

Sometimes the husband's response to his spouse's new attitude is great. We call this the grateful response. In this scenario the wife takes care of him, makes prescribed changes in his diet, walks with him every night. She helps with his medicines, backs off when she has to, and gives him the freedom he needs.

At other times, for the husband, it's the "Oh, my God" response. Here, the guy has a wife who was a pain in the butt before, but now she's mad as hell because he created this can of worms, not her, and she's going to change his life or kill him in the process.

Both of You Are Patients

So there it is. It's incredibly important to realize that there are two patients in the examining room after your husband's chest pain has been diagnosed, not one. It's crucial that everyone—including your husband—understands that you have issues, too, and that they must be dealt with.

As physicians, we recognize that the patient cannot be treated alone. His illness affects his spouse, family, friends, coworkers, and, indeed, the community in which he lives. A diagnosis of heart disease is like throwing a stone into a pond. The waves that move outward represent all the different ways his illness will touch everyone around him.

12

They Didn't Tell Me That . . .

You are now a heart patient. You've had enough tests to last a lifetime. You've had a bypass procedure. You're on new medicines. You've had endless doctor visits, with many more to come. You have new concerns, issues, and fears. Your body feels differently and you are going through new emotions. And you've asked hundreds of questions, many of which were not answered. Many more questions you didn't know how to ask. If your life had problems before, adding heart disease really messes up everything. No one told you that your life was going to be turned upside down—least of all your doctors. This chapter is all about what you can expect and how to deal with a lack of information and a mountain of frustration. It offers a glimpse into your new world and, hopefully, some comfort. You need to know you are not alone, that your issues are not unique, and that you are going to get through it.

An Imperfect System

When you are diagnosed with cardiovascular disease, life as you know it comes to a screeching halt. You have entered a new world—not one you wanted to enter, but here you are. Everything is different. It's overwhelming. You will be unable to hear, absorb, remember, or process all the information you'll be given at the hospital and subsequent visits to the doctor's office. And while you are feeling totally overwhelmed physically and emotionally, many of your medical and personal issues will be overlooked by the medical system. The doctors, nurses, paramedics, technicians, and even the receptionist will leave out very important information you feel you desperately need. These are not bad people; they are doing the best job they can do, but with so many constraints on their time they are simply not going to be able to tell you everything you want to know.

Studies have shown that the amount of information a patient retains from hospital and doctor's visits is directly related to the type of illness you have and how serious it is. For example, if you go to an internist because you have a cold, you will pick up about 70 percent of what you are told. If you go to a cardiologist and are told you have congestive heart failure, not really understanding what that is, you will pick up less than 30 percent of the information.

There is no simple answer, method, or technique to manage all the new demands of heart disease. We believe it is important to understand that there is a common, uniting theme about how our bodies heal and return to health. Recovering from a heart attack or bypass surgery is complicated and involves the whole body. Metaphorically and literally, the heart breaks and needs time to heal and rehabilitate to restore a fully functioning life. It takes six to eight weeks for your heart and body to heal from its initial wounds, and another three to six months of rehab before you'll start feeling good again. Realistically, you are not going to be the same person you were before your heart event, nor should you expect to be. Nonetheless, there is a light at the end of the tunnel. With some hard work and perseverance, you will get through it.

They Didn't Tell Me That . . .

The list below expresses many of the observations and frustrations patients experience during hospital and office visits. Drawn from the experience of our own patients—both men and women—it's a litany of all the things "they" don't tell you, such as:

1. I would have to lie uncomfortably in bed for hours, scared out of my mind in the emergency room, until they figured out what is going on. It's not like in the movies where you walk in, they make a diagnosis, and you are good to go in a matter of minutes.
2. My wife would be ignored throughout the emergency room process.
3. I would be awake during the angiogram.
4. I would feel pain in my groin during and after the angiogram.
5. I would not get out of bed for twelve hours after the angiogram.
6. I would have short-term memory loss issues for up to three to six months after the bypass.

7. After the bypass, I wouldn't be able to stop crying and I still don't know why.

8. They would cut my chest in half.

9. I would be aghast at the unsightly scar between my breasts (especially when the surgeon says it looks fantastic), or that it would be around for six to eight months and then fade.

10. After a bypass, the incisions in my leg, where they removed the veins, would hurt worse than my chest.

11. No one told me how long my hospital stay would be.

12. I would have tubes sticking out of my chest, and every time I coughed, I would feel them rubbing against my insides.

13. I would be a frightening sight for my young kids—or grandkids—to see after the bypass, and that their visits would be very emotional both for me and for them.

14. It would be painful and difficult to urinate or move my bowels after surgery, and I wouldn't be able to go home until I did both.

15. I would have to use a bedpan while there was another patient in the room, or conversely, that I would be in the room when they used the bedpan and have to be subjected to the odor.

16. My roommate would moan all night.

17. No matter how much you complain, you never get any sleep in the hospital because the staff wakes you up every two hours.

18. My arms would feel worse than my chest from the constant blood draws and blood-pressure checks.

19. I should have gotten my questions ready for the doctor's three-minute visits, while I was lying in bed waiting for him all day, but my wife and I never knew when he would show up.

20. After surgery (or other procedures), no food would taste right, or how long this would last.

21. How fatigued I would be after bypass surgery or even after an angioplasty.

22. I was going to bruise or bleed for no discernible cause. Even if I brushed against a wall or an object, my arm would turn blue.

23. My arms would look as though I had been beaten. (This is especially true for older patients who have very thin skin and who bruise easily.)

24. My legs would turn blue after an angioplasty.

25. There would be a lump the size of a dime in my groin from a closure device (a plug that closes the hole in the artery made during an angiogram and remains in place for three to six months as it dissolves).

26. With a medicine called amiodarone commonly used to help control heart rate, my skin would turn gray or that I could not be exposed to the sun while I was taking it. When I play golf, I have to be covered from head to toe with sunblock protection.

27. I wouldn't be able to sleep on my side for a month after a bypass.

28. I wouldn't be able to raise my arm for about a week after having a pacemaker implanted.

29. A pacemaker would protrude from under my skin for up to four months after it was put in. (This is more important for women because a bra strap lies on top of the pacemaker, causing additional discomfort.)

30. My skin at the site of the scar would be so sensitive after a bypass.

31. I would feel terrible for a whole year after a bypass.

32. I would feel so tired for so long for up to a year after a bypass.

33. I might feel dizzy, throw up, and pass out if I take an ACE inhibitor (a medicine that controls blood pressure)—and that every time I get out of bed or a chair I could feel dizzy for a few seconds.

34. I would have no sexual desire for months, and when I finally did my wife would be so afraid about the possible strain on my heart—or even touching me—that we would have no sex.

35. My spouse would look at me differently and feel angry and frustrated because now I have a disease. I don't understand this; after all, I'm the patient.

36. I can't lift more than ten pounds for a month. That means I can't pick up my kids. When they cry in the middle of the night, I have to wake up my wife and she has to get up and take care of them.

37. I would be short of breath after my procedure or what I should do if I also have more chest pain. Does this mean I'm having another heart attack or need another bypass? Do I have to go to the emergency room? Is this a normal part of the healing process?

38. My heart surgeon would lose all interest in me as a patient after I left the hospital.

39. How overwhelmed my spouse and I would be after either a bypass or angioplasty procedure.

40. How I was expected to lose forty pounds, stop smoking, eat better, exercise, and decrease my stress all at the same time.

41. I could not return to work until the doctor gave me a note. I would feel like I was back in school, and without any control over my life.

42. I can only work part-time the first week back at my job, and that I would be totally exhausted.

43. I would wake up the first morning at home, eat breakfast, then feel exhausted and need to take a nap. (Am I ninety years old? I had a bypass; I should be fine.) I wouldn't know my level of immobility. Is this normal after the procedure?

44. I couldn't drive for four to six weeks after my bypass.

45. If I had a pacemaker, it would set off the security alarm at the local clothing store and embarrass the hell out of me when I showed them the card that says I have a pacemaker and still have to take my shirt (or blouse) off and show my scar.

46. What I was supposed to do when I got home. I am now sitting at home, looking at my spouse, who is looking at me. We are both looking at the four walls, and we don't know what to do.

47. How we cope with each other in our new roles. My spouse does the driving, tells me what to eat, tells me not to walk upstairs, tells me we are not having sex, and on top of it, she treats me like a china doll. I have no control. Our roles have changed.

48. I have to ride as a passenger in the car. "They" don't understand that it's more stressful for me when my wife drives. Why can't I drive?

49. Once I had my procedure, I would walk out the door and I'd be done. Or that I was going to be on eight different medicines with different dosing schedules—some for a year, some for two years, some for life. I feel like I'm still a patient.

50. I have heart disease. I don't think I do. I came to the doctor because I was playing volleyball and I hurt my shoulder.

51. I would have to stop smoking.

52. I would have to eat better and exercise. I like to eat and I don't like to exercise. I'm fifty years old and I've done pretty well so far. My wife tells me to eat better and exercise, and I tell her my doctor didn't tell me that.

53. My lifestyle would have to change. I liked my lifestyle and social situation; I like to smoke, drink, and go out with my friends. Now, I have to change all that, or so says my wife.

54. Even if I make all those lifestyle changes, there is a good chance all this might happen again. That the odds are my bypass will last ten years. If I have an angioplasty, it could re-block within the first six months.

55. I have lost control of my life.

56. I can perhaps gain control of my life if I make all the lifestyle modifications I was told to make.

57. My heart disease is never going away. I may be able to get it under control, but it will be with me for the rest of my life.

58. My insurance rates will forever be changed because I have heart disease.

The bottom line is that sometimes the doctors, nurses, and health care professionals you are dealing with sometimes don't give you the proper information, and at other times do, but you don't hear them. But what is important is understanding that being a heart patient is not easy. The only way to get through this is to make sure you get your questions and concerns addressed in a timely fashion. The only bad question is the question not asked or not answered. If your doctor is not addressing your needs, get a new one.

13

The Life of a Cardiac Patient

With all the deep and broad advances that have been made in medicine during the twentieth and twenty-first centuries, none of us expects to get sick, least of all from heart disease. When we do become ill, we expect to be healed quickly and effortlessly. We don't feel like we've signed up for illness, especially a chronic illness like heart disease. So when it does happen, we are not too pleased.

Dealing with illness and chronic disease means you are entering into an unwanted world of inconveniences and unwanted expenses, taking new medicines, undergoing tests and surgical procedures, spending countless hours in waiting rooms, the list goes on. Your complaints, frustration, and fears are real. You are not alone. Pretty much every patient feels the same way. But at the end of the day, you have to get past them. The only one who can improve your life and health is you.

What Our Patients Say

The following is just a representative list of attitudes and complaints heard every day in our clinical practice and should validate patients' fears. Hopefully, this will allow them to accept the inevitability of being sick.

1. I don't like being sick.
2. I don't like feeling tired.
3. I don't like sweating.
4. I don't like the way my heart-healthy food tastes.
5. I don't like this medicine; it leaves a funny aftertaste.
6. I don't like to exercise.
7. I don't like the foods I'm supposed to eat, but I like the foods I'm ordered not to eat, so I eat the foods I shouldn't eat.

8. I don't like waiting in the doctor's office.
9. I don't like spending money on medicines and exercise equipment or athletic club dues.
10. I don't like exercising in front of other people.
11. I don't like my muscles aching.
12. I don't like getting sick (we repeat this because we hear it so much).
13. I don't like people telling me what to do.
14. I don't like my doctor.
15. I don't like people telling me I can't smoke.
16. I don't like having pain in my chest after my bypass operation.
17. I don't like doctors in general; I don't trust them.
18. I don't like hospitals.
19. I don't like tests.
20. I don't like the smell of hospitals; people die in hospitals, so it's the smell of death.
21. I don't like waking up from surgery with a tube sticking out of my nose and mouth and not being able to breathe on my own.
22. I don't like waiting for the results of my tests.
23. I don't like calling the doctor's office and bothering him.
24. I don't like taking time off from work to go to the doctor's office because my life is too important for that.
25. I don't like taking twenty-seven different medicines just for breakfast.
26. I don't like peeing so much.
27. I don't like having difficulty peeing.
28. I don't like not being able to get an erection and I like it even less when I tell the doctor and he says, "You just have to live with it."
29. I don't like complaining to the doctor about the side effects of my medicines and hear him say, "You just have to live with it."
30. I don't like being tired all the time.
31. I don't like going to a cardiac psychologist; I'm not crazy.
32. I don't like having a cardiologist; I don't have a heart problem.
33. I don't like having my wife tell me what to do; I like to be in control.
34. I don't like having my wife drive me in the car; I'm not an invalid.
35. I don't like having my wife tell me I can't lift anything heavier than five pounds.

36. I don't like it when people tell me they know more about my body than I do.
37. I don't like not being in control of my life.
38. I don't like people telling me I can't work.
39. I don't like going back to work and then only working part-time.
40. I don't like people not understanding and appreciating what I'm going through.
41. I don't like people telling me they understand what I'm going through because there is no way in hell they can because I'm going through it and they're not.
42. I don't like thinking about my heart all the time.
43. I don't like worrying about my heart.
44. I don't like waiting for the doctor to call me back.
45. I don't like getting my blood taken, especially when the technician misses on the first two or three or four attempts.
46. I don't like the fact that my blood thinners make me look like I got beat up.

Clearly based on this list, there is plenty not to like about being a heart patient. However, reflecting on this chapter should allow patients to identify their issues and hopefully get past them. It is normal to feel outraged over all the inconveniences of your disease. But by making positive lifestyle choices (such as the ones offered in proceeding chapters), you can feel better and get the most enjoyment and satisfaction from your life.

14

Common Misperceptions

Most people have misperceptions about what defines a healthy life, and more important, about how healthy they truly are. These misperceptions develop from a long history of unhealthy habits and routines. However, they are significant in that they cause medical problems and make them more difficult to solve.

The Dangers of Self-Deception

Over the course of our lives, we have the tendency to develop and even celebrate our own system of core beliefs, perceptions, and habits concerning ourselves and the world that determine how we conduct our lives. Unfortunately, these core beliefs don't always correspond with the optimal way of treating heart disease. In fact, they may be undermining your health and bringing you into a danger zone where you could lose your life. It is not enough to let your cardiologist customize your care while treating your coronary artery disease. You have to step up to the plate and conform to specific treatment paths that will serve you well over the long term. Otherwise, you are in denial and your health will not benefit from keeping your head firmly stuck in the sand.

The transition from "regular life" to "heart-patient life" is not easy or pleasant. The transition to a healthy lifestyle, if you are heart patient, is made all the more difficult if you stubbornly stand by your old beliefs about yourself and what is "healthy." Some common misperceptions—or personal myths—about your health and well-being may include the following:

- I only need six hours of sleep a night.
- People who need lots of sleep are weak or lazy.
- I don't have stress.

- It's OK to have a six-pack of beer every night.
- It's OK to have three martinis every night.
- I'm too busy to exercise.
- I can't quit smoking. It's too hard.
- I don't eat that much; in fact, I eat pretty healthily.
- I can't understand why I gain weight because I eat practically nothing all day.
- I'm too busy to plan my meals.
- I don't have heart disease; in fact, I feel fine.
- It's the doctor's job to cure me; I'm not responsible.
- I'm not supposed to be sick; I don't have the time.
- I know how to handle my stress; it's not a factor for me.
- I can't get my blood pressure under control, but I don't believe it has anything to do with my weight or what I eat. I need a new doctor and new medicines.
- Smoking is not causing my heart problem.
- Of course I ate all six doughnuts in the box; they were fat-free and cholesterol-free.
- I can drink as much caffeine as I want. It doesn't affect me; I'm used to it.
- I can't fall asleep until one or two a.m., but it's not due to the caffeine I drink.
- Although I have headaches five out of seven days a week, it's not due to stress.
- Although I have irritable bowel syndrome, it's not due to stress.
- Although I have stomach ulcers, it's not due to stress.
- I didn't think these meds were working, so I stopped taking them.
- It's OK to only take my medicine when I feel bad.
- Smoking reduces my stress.
- I try to keep my blood sugar around 130; that's good.
- I only need to take my blood pressure medication when I have a headache.
- Doesn't everybody get some chest pain when they exercise?
- I can't bother my doctor about that.
- Doesn't everybody get swollen feet at the end of the day?
- It's normal to get short of breath when you walk up a flight of stairs.

- I don't sleep at night, I'm really irritable, I can't concentrate, and I get panicky, but I'm not depressed or anxious.

If you believe any of these statements, you are deceiving yourself and going in the wrong direction. In fact, you are far away from living a more healthy life with heart disease.

In order for you to get better, you have to first identify the "denials"—all the things you want to believe are healthy and normal about your lifestyle but are actually causing your heart problems. Then run, don't walk, to a cardiac psychologist who is equipped to help you deal with these issues. There is no "pill" or easy fix here. You have to roll up your sleeves and be prepared to put in the time and effort needed to get better and stay well not just today or tomorrow but for the rest of your life.

15

The Statistics Game

Pick up any book that purports to tell you the way to better health and you'll be bombarded with statistics and numbers on every page. Why? Because use of statistics and other medical numbers creates a perception of validity. Although some data may be helpful, they are often misleading and misinterpreted. Medical statistics can lead the patient and the general population to confusion. In some cases, statistics can actually steer people down the wrong path. This is as common to heart disease as any other illness and needs to be cleared up.

Numbers Don't Tell the Whole Story

Our society is flooded with medical statistics and "factoids" that pour of out of self-help books, newspaper articles, magazines, TV, and the Internet. Even though these numbers are everywhere and seemingly impossible to escape, our advice is to take them with a big grain of salt. Don't get overly caught up in them, and, more important, don't make serious lifestyle changes that are solely based on information from the mass media. If you do find a convincing piece of information or statistic that speaks to you, talk to a doctor or health-care professional whose opinion you trust and who can help you determine the validity of a statistic or other information before you act on it.

The facts and statistics surrounding breast cancer provide a good illustration of our admonition. The very thought of breast cancer evokes images of pain, suffering, humiliation, and early death. Ask a woman what disease she is most afraid of and she will almost always say breast cancer. But statistical evidence says that the average woman has a one in twenty-five risk of dying of breast cancer* but a one in two risk of dying from heart disease.** If this is true, then why are more women concerned about breast cancer than about heart disease?

The answer is the breast cancer lobby has done a terrific job of educating the public about the dangers of breast cancer, the benefits of early detection, and improvements in breast cancer procedures, medications, and recovery. We are not implying that their efforts are misleading; what we are saying is that what you hear, read, and are exposed to, while it may be accurate, may not necessarily apply to you. Our advice is: Don't let a statistic dictate what you should be worried about. Instead, you need to work with your doctor to figure out what your risks are, based on your own medical history and that of your family. For example, a fifty-eight-year-old woman with a history of high blood pressure, smoking, high cholesterol, too much weight, and a mother and sister who died from heart attacks in their sixties should make investigating heart disease her first priority, while also making sure to be screened for breast cancer.

What Do Percentages Really Tell You?

Another example of numbers telling us incomplete stories is the statistics we so often read in books or magazines about a treatment or a "new medicine that can lower your risk of heart disease by 25 percent." But what does that really mean? Twenty-five percent of what? Does this mean you have a 75 percent chance of dying if you don't take the medicine? Or that you will live 25 percent longer than you would have if you do take the medicine?

The truth is we don't know—and can't know—because the percentage tells us nothing specifically about you. The numbers are all about convincing you that if you take the medicine, you may have a lower chance of having another heart problem. What is never explained or provided in the statistic or factoid is that the medicine must be taken under very specific circumstances to be effective and in order to achieve the desired medical benefits. The best dosage, age, and gender groups to whom the medication applies, and whether or not other medications or medical problems may counteract the medication are not explained either.

*American Cancer Society. *Breast Cancer Facts and Figures 2005–2006*. Atlanta, GA, 2005.

**ACC/AHA 2007 Guidelines, *Update for the Diagnosis and Management of Chronic Heart Failure in the Adult* (American College of Cardiology Foundation and American Heart Association, Inc.).

Be careful how you interpret percentages, because they can be misleading. For example, take a study that compares one hundred people who eat Brussels sprouts with another one hundred people who don't. One person in the Brussels sprouts–eating group has a heart attack, while two people in the non-Brussels sprouts–eating group have heart attacks: the difference is one person. The study, however, will claim the risk reduction from eating Brussels sprouts is 50 percent (one divided by the two). But in reality only one more person had a heart attack in the non-Brussels sprout–eating group. Thus, the "true" risk reduction is quite minor, but the statistic would lead you to believe otherwise.

Once again, we can't argue strongly enough for using medical statistics and factoids wisely. All medical information should be discussed and analyzed with your health-care professional before you make any medical or lifestyle change that is based on a statistic.

PART III

Cardiac Psychology and Treatment

The essence of successful treatment of coronary artery disease is not to try to do everything at once. This approach is destined for failure. You can't stop smoking, lose forty pounds, completely revamp your diet, start exercising, get eight hours of sleep every night, and cut back on stress all at the same time. It just won't happen. At the end of the day, however, you have to make these changes to restore the health of your heart.

The key to an effective treatment program is to first figure out what the key issues are for each patient. You need to identify your specific issues in order to know what to change. No two patients are alike. Here is where a cardiac psychologist comes in.

Every person who has coronary artery disease has behaviors that must be modified; otherwise, he or she wouldn't be a cardiac patient. Often patients don't want to accept the fact that their behaviors are the cause of their heart disease. The cardiac psychologist works with each individual patient to determine the necessary strategies for change. Everybody has different strengths and limitations. The cardiac psychologist first helps the patient understand what behaviors need changing; second, decides the sequence of change; and third, implements the plan. It is an intense, focused, result-oriented process.

If seeing a cardiac psychologist is so important, why isn't every cardiac patient referred to one? The answer is two-fold: First, many doctors and patients don't even know that cardiac psychologists exist. And second, truthfully, both doctors and patients find it easier to give and take a pill rather than deal with the underlying lifestyle behaviors that need to be changed such as smoking, obesity, stress, and exercise. We believe that every cardiac patient should see a cardiac psychologist for at least an initial assessment. In all likelihood you will have to push your doctor for a referral to see one.

To explain what the cardiac psychologist does, Part III contains an open, no-bull discussion of stress reduction, smoking cessation, exercise, diet, and weight management. To bring the discussion home, we also tell you how the eight cardiac patients in Part I were treated and how they are faring in recovery.

16 | Motivating One Life Change at a Time

Successfully treating the post-procedural cardiac patient involves four major lifestyle changes: stress, diet, smoking, and exercise. We focus on one behavior at a time because, let's be honest, if you try to do more than one, it works for about two days. Critical to treatment is to first find the hook—the why, the motivating factor—that makes each patient understand that he or she needs to make the necessary lifestyle changes.

Getting Real about Recovery

Most cardiac patients don't understand that they must make certain behavioral changes if they do not want to enter the revolving door of visiting the cardiologist again and again and undergoing repeated procedures.

Cardiac patients must also understand that they need help, sometimes a little, sometimes a lot, in changing these behaviors. They cannot do it alone; they need direction. This is where cardiac psychology comes in. A cardiac psychologist will work with the patient and his or her family and help them formulate and implement a plan for treating one or more of the four key issues that lie at the heart of heart disease: stress, diet, smoking, and exercise.

Three elements are critical to the plan: treating one lifestyle change at a time, helping the patient maintain positive change over time, and finding the patient's own specific hook for change.

What's the hook?

Simply put, a hook gives the patient the why—why he or she has to get better and make the change. If it sounds like a motivating factor, it is. The key is to find the right motivating factor for you—and then use it.

Here's an example of the necessity of finding a hook and how tricky it can be to stick with it. A patient comes in to the doctor's office after experiencing a heart attack. She has coronary disease and has had an angioplasty. The doctor needs to convince the patient that because she has high cholesterol, she must lose weight, eat better, and stop smoking. In addition, she has to control her anxiety and sleep better. But just telling the patient everything she has to do all at once usually doesn't cut it. Believe it or not, the fact that she has heart disease and almost died from it may not necessarily motivate her to make serious changes. The entire medical team (cardiologist, clinical psychologist, internist, nurse, technician) often has to help a patient find the motivating force, or hook, to make changes one at a time and then help the patient stick with them.

In our practice we have found the following hooks to be particularly powerful motivators that have lead to positive and lasting changes. Here are a few of the hooks:

- Getting control of your life back.
- Fear of having another heart attack.
- Fear of having another heart surgery.
- Fear of dying.
- Fear of disability.
- Wanting less pain—in your knees, back, hips, feet, body.
- Being able to get down on the floor and play with your grandchildren.
- Pride of proving something to somebody.
- Avoiding embarrassment, such as a public heart attack.
- Being afraid to lose the ability to care for your family.
- Wanting to be with your family; not wanting to die at a young age.
- Validation—getting someone to care.
- Feeling better.
- Vanity—pride in how you look.
- Competition—pride at winning.
- Making someone proud of you.
- Money—loss of earning potential.
- A class reunion.
- Getting off your medicines.

- Fear of failure.
- Disappointment in yourself.
- Getting better to have sex again.
- Getting into smaller-size clothes.
- Being able to breathe again.
- Shopping in normal-size stores vs. Big and Tall.
- Being able to golf, garden, or walk farther than one hundred feet without gasping for air.
- Being able to face the relatives at the next holiday gathering.
- Being sick and tired of being sick and tired.
- Fed up with freezing when standing outside to have a smoke.
- Tired of stomach pains from stress.
- Tired of chronic headaches from stress.
- Tired of having panic attacks.
- Tired of having chest pains from stress.
- Your doctor "told you to." (On the surface, this may not look like much of a hook, but the truth is what a doctor tells you to do can be a very powerful motivational force).

People often have more than one hook, which may change over time. However, focusing on what a patient wants now and is willing to do to improve his or her life is the key. A good cardiac health-care team, which at a minimum should include a cardiologist and cardiac psychologist, will work together to identify and implement the best strategies to get their patient healthier.

17

The Core of Heart Disease: Stress

Stress is not just another issue a cardiac psychologist deals with when treating heart disease patients. Stress is the root cause of all the other exacerbating problems: bad diet, smoking, lack of exercise. The cardiologist will treat high blood pressure, high cholesterol, and blocked arteries with medicines and angioplasty. But the major critical issue for most of our heart problems is stress—the everyday habitual grind, pressures, and struggles of life. The goal of the cardiac psychologist is to identify the patient's key stressors and then turn that stress into something manageable.

The Biggest Killer

Nothing affects our health and wreaks more havoc on our body and mind—whether it's our heart, digestive system, kidneys, joints, back, head, or psyche—than stress. Stress causes heart disease, ulcers, irritable bowel disorder, chronic fatigue, body pain, rashes, teeth grinding, and sleep problems. We are so used to feeling stressed that we forget what it feels like not to be stressed. "Feeling good" now comes in a pint of ice cream, stuffing ourselves until we're numb, sitting on the couch until we fall asleep, or having a cigarette. For many, any feeling of well-being has long been gone.

Truthfully, stress is killing us. Here are some facts that may provide a little perspective on stress:

- In the United States we are working harder and longer hours every year—on average fifty hours per week, which is a ten-hour workday.*

---

*Al Gini, *My Job, My Self: Work and the Creation of the Modern Individual* (New York, Routledge, 2000), 75–87.

- We average just under two hours commuting per day, making it a twelve-hour workday.
- We take fewer than ten days of paid vacation per year.
- Most of us awake before six a.m. and get home after six p.m. each day.
- When we come home from that long workday and onerous commute, we eat enough food for a week, struggle mightily to spend some quality time with our also stressed family members, and eventually fall asleep in front of the TV between eleven p.m. and midnight.
- We are sleep-deprived, overcaffeinated, and overscheduled.
- We're in greater financial debt than ever.

It should therefore be no surprise that we also have the highest rate of heart disease in the world, and our stressful, overcrammed lives are the direct cause. Our stressful lives result in poor eating habits, participation in less and less physical activity, and sleep deprivation. Getting less than seven hours of sleep per night increases your craving for sugar and diminishes your feeling of fullness after eating. Sleep deprivation also makes you irritable, anxious, and depressed, and impairs your attention and concentration.

Clearly, stress causes a downward spiral that takes a negative toll on all aspects of life, especially our health. When you learn how to better control, manage, and decrease your stress, you can begin to create an upward spiral that positively improves the health of your heart and overall quality of life.

When you visit your doctor with a health complaint, the most unsatisfactory diagnosis you're likely to hear is that the cause of your medical problem is stress. In fact, you may feel that your doctor is being dismissive and not taking your problems seriously when he or she gives you this diagnosis. You want to be given a prescription or some other remedy to make your medical problems go away, because this is what we are all programmed to expect. And in many instances, medical treatment works. However, it rarely lasts. Why? Because the real problem hasn't been addressed.

As your ailment keeps returning and you grow more frustrated with your doctor, your treatment, and yourself, you get desperate and extreme in treating your problems—with more doctors, more meds, and more tests. The truth is that stress, and nothing else, is the culprit for most of our medical problems, barring rare and early age-onset diseases. People don't want to hear that their overscheduled, stressful lives are at the root of their medical problems because it's like telling them to control the weather, a seemingly impossible feat. Patients simply want to feel better and make their problems go away—Doctor, give me another pill! In short, you want your symptoms treated because it's a hell of a lot easier than dealing with the root causes.

What Exactly Is Stress?

Stress is any force that produces strain on our bodies and minds. Stress is about our struggles, fears, frustrations, and life's pressures, problems, and threats. What exactly does stress do? It has a real impact on our hearts and bodies. Prolonged stress increases levels of adrenaline, causing elevated blood pressure and heart rate. Chronic elevated blood pressure wears out your heart and damages your coronary arteries, resulting in heart disease and strokes.

Prolonged stress also increases your levels of cortisol, a naturally produced steroid. High levels of cortisol lead to an increase in blood sugar, diabetes, high blood pressure, decreases in bone density, decreases in muscle tissue, increased abdominal fat, blood-clotting disorders, and heart disease. High levels of cortisol also suppress your immune system, leading to infection and chronic fatigue.

Ongoing, daily stress is very real and needs to be dealt with aggressively. Stress can be superficial or deep-rooted, and it can be related, among many other causes, to:

- Too many demands on your life.
- Your job, finances, or marriage.
- Taking care of children and/or elderly parents.
- A long commute.
- An annoying neighbor.
- A messy house, late payments, general disorganization.
- Chronic pain or chronic medical problems.
- Feelings of inadequacy, failure, or low self-esteem.
- Long-standing anger issues.
- A childhood trauma—sexual, physical, emotional, or mental—that has never been dealt with.

Although most doctors can detect when a patient is feeling stressed, most don't know how to effectively treat it, either because they don't have the time or are not comfortable telling the patient that his or her problem is stress related. So the patient gets treated for the stomach pain, or the headaches, or the sleep problems, or the high blood pressure with another pill.

A cardiologist will often send a patient back to an internist or primary-care doctor to address any non-heart issues, particularly if they are psychological or emotional. Cardiologists are often unwilling to tell patients that stress is a factor because they are afraid their patients will think they're being told that they're crazy.

The Cardiac Psychologist's Role

The tag-team approach of a cardiologist and cardiac psychologist enables cardiologists to more comfortably and confidently refer their patients to a person specifically trained to assess and treat stress. Often, the patient does not expect this, but that's what's needed. The cardiologist has to explain to the patient and make them understand that their stress is a critical part of their medical problem and that their stress is causing them to smoke, overeat, have high blood pressure, elevated heart rates, elevated blood sugar, and lose sleep—the other direct causes of heart disease.

Although most heart patients know stress is bad, most of them are reluctant to do anything about it. Here's why:

- They don't think they're stressed.
- They accept their level of misery.
- They don't believe they can alter their stress level.
- They want to stop stressing but don't know where to start.
- They're afraid of failing.
- By admitting they have stress, they're admitting weakness.
- It's too much work to deal with stress.
- They and their family have become comfortable with the stress. They think they're handling it well.
- They believe it is more stressful to accept, deal with, and change the stress in their lives than it is to simply live with it.

The Stress Test

If you still don't believe that stress is an issue in your life, please take the following test. Put a check mark by any question that you would answer with a "yes."

_____ Do you have money problems?

_____ Do you have job dissatisfaction?

_____ Do you dislike your boss?

_____ Do you dislike your coworkers?

_____ Are you a caretaker of a relative?

_____ Have you lost your job?

_____ Do you have marital problems?

_____ Are you getting a divorce?

_____ Are you just getting over a divorce?

_____ Are you and your spouse separated?

_____ Are you involved in a lawsuit?

_____ Has anybody recently moved into or out of your house? Children? A parent?

_____ Are you moving?

_____ Have you been fired?

_____ Do you feel trapped in your job?

_____ Do you have chronic sleep problems?

_____ Do you have a chronic pain problem?

_____ Do you have issues regarding your children's education, physical health, or mental health?

_____ Do you have health care insurance problems?

_____ Do you have medical problems?

_____ Do you have sibling rivalry issues?

_____ Has a loved one recently died?

_____ Are you dealing with a family member's estate?

_____ Is someone telling you to quit smoking, eat better, or exercise more?

It's very easy to score the test. Count the number of items you checked, multiply this by 3.72, divide by 6.5, find the square root, and then throw the whole thing out because if you said yes to even one of the questions, you are stressed.

If your problems are not going away any time soon, then you may need help to better deal with them—or your health will suffer.

What to Expect from Your Cardiac Psychologist

While most doctors will recognize that a patient's stress is negatively impacting his or her life, most of them do not refer the patient to a cardiac psychologist for further evaluation and treatment. The lucky ones who are referred and are willing to try it out, can expect the following:

For the first time, you will have a well-trained health-care professional who is taking the time—forty-five to sixty minutes a session—to listen, understand, and not judge you, your struggles, or where you are coming from. Perhaps the most valuable treatment your cardiac psychologist can give you is hope and the reassurance that you are not alone, and that your health and life can improve.

Your cardiac psychologist will give you an individual evaluation and therapy plan. He or she will help you identify stressors, understand how stress is involved in your ill health, and help you begin to manage that stress. He or she will help you become less emotionally reactive. The goal is to improve your coping skills designed to decrease the level of your worry, anxiety, anger, and even loneliness. In short, you will be taught skills to control the stressors in your life instead of giving them all the control.

Stress Management—The Key to Heart Health

Stress can be a very complicated issue because it has multiple layers like an onion. Stress management must be tailored to fit the individual for the simple reason that it is different for every patient. Stress cannot be dealt with in three or five steps, or in the twenty generalized steps that so many stress management books set out. Few, if any, of these easy formulas can address your specific and individual issues, such as long-standing marital problems or family, money, and parenting dilemmas. Nor can any self-help book do a comprehensive job of mitigating a history of trauma and abuse. These issues are far too complicated to be fixed by any catchall program, and we are not offering one here, either.

Managing and decreasing stress, however, can be accomplished by doing any one or all four of the following:

1. Increasing your awareness by learning how to live and consciously experience the present moment.
2. Learning "conscious breathing," taking relaxation training, or learning how to meditate.
3. Decreasing your negativity (pessimism and worry) by altering your thinking, your language, and gaining a healthier perspective.
4. Getting more rest and sleep.

The goal of stress management is to train your mind and body to be less reactive, thereby lowering your stress hormones, adrenaline and cortisol. Emotions such as worry, anger, hostility, and despair elevate these hormones, which places strain on your heart by increasing your heart rate and blood pressure. Experiencing these emotions for short durations such as hours or even a day is normal and not harmful. But longer durations, days on end, means that you are putting your heart at risk.

But first, a quick note about personality types—a collection of normal human traits that have been categorized by scientists as type A, type B, type C, and type D. Over the past forty years, research has studied the relationship between these four personality types and elevated risk for heart disease. Initially, it was discovered that men with type-A personalities—typically men who are impatient, highly competitive, assertive, and incapable of relaxation—were more likely to have heart attacks and be diagnosed with heart disease as compared to men who are less likely to exhibit those behavior patterns. However, further research demonstrated that type-A personality was not the culprit. Rather, the key emotion linked to heart disease was hostility. People who are hostile—that is, commonly express anger, blame others for their problems, and never take responsibility for their decisions—were the ones with higher rates of heart disease. Researchers also discovered that type-D personalities—people whose

Personality Types and Their Characteristics

A *type-A* person is impatient, highly competitive, more assertive, and incapable of relaxation.

A *type-B* person is relaxed and noncompetitive.

A *type-C* person is pleasant, avoids conflict, and suppresses feelings.

A *type-D* person is anxious, irritable, and socially inhibited.

behavior patterns exhibit anxiety, worry, and irritability, and who are socially inhibited—appear to have a higher incidence of heart disease. No similar link was found for type-B and type-C personalities. However, recent research and clinical evidence support the theory that experiencing certain emotions such as hostility, anxiety, and hopelessness over the long term has a more harmful effect on heart health than any specific "personality type." Efforts to mitigate these negative emotions—which are all stress emotions—through stress management training, assertiveness training, psychotherapy, and exercise are key to lowering the risk of heart disease and improving health.

Increasing Awareness

Increasing awareness is the critical link in the chain of events that enables you to gain control over your life and heart health. Conscious awareness is the starting point by which you can be in control of your emotions, thoughts, and behaviors that will ultimately help to heal the body.

In simple terms, increasing or elevating your awareness is like showing up to every exam you've ever had to take in your life and knowing that no matter how well you do, it will be OK. You have more peace and confidence. Contrast this feeling to taking a final exam unprepared and fearing the outcome. Increasing awareness, learning how to live and experience the moment, is by definition more peaceful. Why? Because the only place you can ever truly be is where you are.

Personalities, Negative Emotions, Stress, and Heart Disease

Specific personalities do not cause heart attacks or heart disease. However, chronic experience of negative emotions such as hostility, anxiety, and hopelessness appears to be linked with heart disease. Commonly people with high levels of stress are indeed feeling a combination of these emotions. The exact biochemical relationship between stress, negative emotions, and heart disease is not fully understood. However, there is evidence that chronically elevated levels of adrenaline and cortisol due to stress is bad news for the heart and body because these hormones elevate blood pressure, suppress the immune system, tax the thyroid gland, deregulate insulin and blood sugar, and are responsible for higher levels of inflammatory chemicals in the blood. The good news is that decreasing and leveling off adrenaline and cortisol (in other words, decreasing stress) through relaxation, laughter, optimism, and improved communication may indeed mitigate heart problems and give people the control to improve their health and lives.

Even if you don't like where you are, the better you get at living in the moment the better you will feel. By accepting what is, your negative feelings begin to dissolve and the tension in your mind and body diminish, lowering stress hormones and lessoning the strain on your heart.

It's completely normal to revisit the past and anticipate what might happen in the future. But if you spend too much time thinking about and emotionally reacting to events that either no longer exist (the past), or have not yet happened (the future), you can get stuck in state of worry and regret that stresses you out and, consequently, increases the levels of adrenaline and cortisol in your system. The minute you focus your thoughts on the moment and keep them in the present, those levels drop. Remember, chronically elevated levels of adrenaline and cortisol place strain on the heart by increasing heart rate, blood pressure, and blood sugar levels, which increases the risk of heart disease. A wonderful, yet simple technique is to say and repeat the lyrics to the late, great Marvin Gaye's song "What's Going On." Do this and your stress will go down, as well as the level of adrenaline and cortisol in your system. The stress in your life won't be entirely eliminated, but it will decrease. Other phrases or sayings that might help to get and keep you in the moment are, "Right now is perfect; it is all I will ever have," "If not now, when?," and "Just pay attention."

The more conscious time you spend in the moment, the better you will feel. By being in the moment, you can now deal with your problems and your anxiety and, most important, appreciate when good things happen.

If you are too busy thinking about the future, you run the risk of skipping right by the good things in the present. A technique to help you increase awareness is to focus more on your senses—on smells,

Techniques for Being in the Moment

Nothing in our culture fosters or nurtures being in the moment. We are bombarded and marketed to death with images and sounds influencing us to want more, more, more. The chase becomes an addiction. Our thoughts and consciousness are in a constant state of wanting something other than where we are and what we have. Meditation, relaxation training, yoga, and tai chi are just a few techniques that can help bring you into the moment. Most local fitness centers, YMCAs, spas, and yoga studios offer classes and groups that can teach you how to increase awareness and ultimately lower stress. Participation in these classes either in a group or on an individual basis can truly change your life.

sights, sounds, tastes, and tactile sensations. Learn to taste every bite you take, really listen to music as opposed to just hearing it in the background, and focus on the way a breeze feels on your skin. There are countless other simple sensations you can experience every day that can keep you in the moment. The more time you spend there, the more quickly you will let go of the stresses in your life.

Conscious Breathing

Learn to take conscious breaths throughout the day. When you take in a full breath and, upon exhaling, let your body flop and relax, like a sigh, this lowers adrenaline and cortisol, thus decreasing blood pressure and heart rate. Efforts to control and lower blood pressure are critical to minimizing the risk for heart disease and stroke. If you sigh two to five times at a time, and do it ten times a day, you will immediately feel better. Do this for a week or longer and your whole body will feel better. You will also find it increasingly easier to handle everyday stress. If you can practice meditation, relaxation techniques, yoga, tai chi, or simply exercise daily, your mind, body, and health will greatly improve. In the meantime, put sticky notes around your house, car, and workplace with the word "breathe" on them. Every time you see the note, take a breath. Your stress will begin to melt away.

Decrease Negativity

Letting go of negative self-talk is a wonderful stress-reducing method. Let go of constant worry, anger, pessimism, and self-doubt. These emotions are maintained and fueled by our own internal dialogue and it's eating you alive. Some people love to worry or be angry, but that's a separate problem. Most people, however, get tired of being in a constant state of anxiety and irritability. A method to decrease negativity is to change the language you use to communicate with other people as well as the way you think about yourself. When our language and internal dialogue change, our emotions change.

It is enormously common for people to have childhood memories that are ingrained in their being. These memories are based on experiences with family members, parents, siblings, teachers, coaches, and religious leaders. Unfortunately for many, the memories of what others have said and done often become negative and painful internal recordings that are played over and over again and that strongly influence how we think and feel. These internal recordings might include messages such as "You will never amount to anything," "You have such a pretty face, too bad you can't lose the weight," "How come you can't be as smart as your sister or brother?" and "I know you try, but once again it is not good enough." It is apparent that long-standing negative input can have a long-term negative impact.

Fortunately, most of us have had positive influences growing up that provide a counterbalance to any negative experiences. But for some people, negative and painful experiences are dominant, resulting in an abundance of overlearned and rehearsed negative thoughts, language, and feelings. The goal is to replace negative and all-or-nothing words and phrases, such as "never," "always," "everything," "I know what's going to happen," "I'm a failure," "He/she is a failure," and "It won't work," with more realistic, balanced, and positive language, such as "maybe," "We'll see," "Let's try again," "It could be worse," "You never know," "I can do it," and "I'm not perfect, nor will I try to be." By eliminating and replacing negative language, your mood, attitude, and stress levels will improve.

Perspective

Most of our problems are simply negative interpretations and reactions to minor issues. Other than a truly serious crisis such as the death of a loved one, divorce, job loss, or being given the news of a deadly diagnosis, most of our daily stress is in fact minor. Ninety-nine percent of our day, week, month, and year is filled with minor issues, annoyances, and conflicts. However, we act as though everyday minor problems are as serious as major problems. Although it may be inevitable that a very stressful and serious event will happen once or twice a year, we can choose not to respond to minor daily events as if the sky is falling.

When you begin to alter language and, through your own thoughts, transform "doom" to "opportune," your stress will go down. When you gain perspective and choose not to get lost in overcharged responses to minor issues, your stress goes down. This is not just positive thinking; it's taking ownership of your thoughts, language, and reactions, which can then be transformed.

You can start your day by thinking and saying, "It's going to stink." Or you can announce that you are going to "find a way to make it work—I'll do my best, which will have to be good enough." Your stress, adrenaline and cortisol levels, and blood pressure will all go down immediately by using more balanced and opportunistic language. The day is coming fast, so enjoy the moment, take a breath, and say, "I'll figure it out; I always do."

There are thousands of techniques people use to reduce stress. Some are heart healthy, such as taking walks, playing chess, reading, bowling, working in the garage, gardening, and meditation, while others, such as overeating, smoking, alcohol abuse, and yelling, are not. If you are focusing your life and attention on activities and thoughts that bring serenity, peace, creativity, passion, laughter, and hope, you are clearly moving in the right direction.

The Importance of Sleep and Rest

Our nation is desperately sleep deprived. We are sleeping less and less. It has become a badge of honor for many to let friends and business associates know how little sleep they need. Unfortunately, people who give sleep short shrift are fools but don't know it. The fact is 90 percent of all the adults on the planet require a minimum of eight hours of quality sleep each night to maintain our health and daily energy needs. Less than that and our bodies will suffer. Our busy, overscheduled lifestyles and incredibly unhealthy nighttime sleep habits such as falling asleep in front of the TV and overeating before getting into bed contribute to later and later sleep times and earlier awakenings. Simply put, if you are consistently getting less than seven hours of sleep per night your body is getting beat up.

You may be accustomed to five or six hours of sleep per night, but this is equivalent to walking up hill all day long. Over time, your body will wear down. Sleep deprivation results in lower energy, poorer concentration, suppressed immune system, sugar cravings, weight gain, irritability, depression, anxiety, and an overtaxed ability to cope with life. In addition, sleep deprivation contributes to elevated levels of

A Note on Coffee and Caffeine

Generally, one cup of coffee a day is OK. Be careful, though, most people have "portion distortion"—a ten-, twelve-, sixteen-, or twenty-ounce cup is not a "normal" cup. An eight-ounce cup of coffee has on average 120 milligrams of caffeine. A good rule is to stay under 200 milligrams of caffeine per day—more than that will overly crank your adrenaline and cortisol levels. Most twelve-ounce soda drinks and tea have a little less than half the caffeine of coffee.

Turn Off the Tube

Many people like falling asleep with the TV in the background because it helps them not think about anything. The problem is, even with your eyes closed, the flickering light continues to stimulate your optic nerve, making it more difficult for you to fall into deep, restorative sleep. People claim that if they don't have the TV on when they are lying in bed, their minds will race and they'll start worrying about life, preventing them from falling asleep faster. But faster sleep does not equal better sleep. If you wouldn't put your baby or young child in front of a TV at bedtime, why should you sabotage your own sleep this way?

adrenaline and cortisol that put you at risk for numerous medical problems, above all, heart disease. And to make matters worse, many people overcaffeinate themselves with coffee and soda to compensate for their low energy and fatigue. Heavy doses of caffeine, like sleep deprivation, also increase adrenaline and cortisol, which is a significant health risk.

In short, getting more sleep and rest improves your energy, mood, attitude, feeling of well-being, immune system, and ability to manage stress and daily life.

Our sleep habits can be nightmarishly (pun intended) complex. The combination of getting to bed too late, falling asleep with the TV, too much caffeine in the day and night, overeating at night, improper use of sleep medications, overactive bladders, middle-of-the-night awakenings, difficulty falling back asleep in the middle of the night, insomnia, and sleep breathing disorders like sleep apnea (which contributes to poor sleep quality) are all impacting our ability to get a decent, restful night's sleep.

The key point is that you need more sleep and rest. There are countless books on sleep that enumerate various disorders and provide detailed methods to improve your sleep. Here are a few simple but key recommendations that will improve your sleep quantity and quality very quickly.

1. Wind down one hour before bedtime. Do some light reading, watch a little TV, or take a shower or bath. Don't start doing chores, reading e-mail, and getting busy.
2. Get into bed ten to thirty minutes earlier than your "normal" time.
3. Understand that is normal to take ten to thirty minutes to fall asleep.
4. Darken your room as much as possible.
5. If you wake up in the middle of the night and can't get back to sleep

within thirty minutes, get out of bed and do some light reading in dim light until you are drowsy again. Then get back into bed and try to fall back asleep.

6. Push your wake-up time ten to thirty minutes later. Get creative and figure out how to get to work a little later or cut back on your morning routine.

7. Don't have any caffeine after two o'clock in the afternoon.

8. Don't have a big meal or lots of liquids later than two hours before bed. Have only a small snack before bed, such as a small bowl of cereal or four ounces of a beverage.

9. A ten- to thirty-minute midday nap can be as refreshing as a cold glass of water on a hot summer day.

10. Finally, if you take sleep medication, work with your doctor to develop a regimented medication plan where you take the medication at the same time every night for a definitive time period. Then reevaluate taking the medication.

The important thing is to start following as many of these recommendations as possible. If you make improving your sleep a priority, your health and your life will noticeably and significantly improve.

18

Walk and Your Heart Walks with You

Exercise is all about lifestyle and attitude. It's critical for your heart and health. To many people it's an annoying activity that is best avoided. For others, it can be an enjoyable, positive, life-altering experience. Either way, exercise is critical. It decreases the risk of getting heart disease and the risk of recurrence once you have it.

Exercise Is a Choice

The number one reason why people don't exercise is because they simply don't want to. It's not laziness; it's not physical limitation; it's not because of time constraints—don't fool yourself. Although most people understand how important exercise is to their health, given the choice between exercising and going about their daily routine, they choose not to alter their routine.

Here is a meaningful statistic: Only about 11 percent of the people in this country exercise daily, and only 20 percent exercise more than three times a week for a reasonable length of time.* Here are some often-heard reasons why some of our patients avoid exercising:

"It's just not my thing."
"It hurts."
"It's embarrassing."
"I don't know what to do. I've never really exercised before."
"It makes me feel tired the rest of the day."
"It might damage my heart even further."
"I don't like to sweat."
"It's not fun; it's boring."

* United Press International Poll: Most Have Exercise Regime, 2007.

"I don't like health clubs."

"I don't have the time" is the excuse we hear most frequently, and it's totally unacceptable. Managing time is not the issue here; it's about managing choices. We know people have very busy schedules. They have major responsibilities—they work, they have families, they have social obligations—but, truly, it's a matter of choice, not time. Anything you want to do, or have to do, you will find time for. Either you figure out a way to move your body on a regular basis or you don't. Although walking your dog is moving your body, and while it's great for your dog, it doesn't provide enough meaningful exercise for you. And the same goes for walking nine or eighteen holes of golf. Sorry about that!

You have to make a conscious choice and effort to exercise. If you don't, you are launching yourself down a path fraught with tremendous medical risks and disabilities, affecting not only your life but your family's. Exercise:

- decreases stress.
- boosts energy.
- helps you sleep better.
- helps you eat less and eat healthier food.
- helps you get stronger.
- increases endurance.
- improves mood.
- improves your sex life.
- strengthens your heart.
- decreases blood pressure.
- decreases heart rate.
- decreases cholesterol.
- decreases the risk of having a heart attack.
- decreases risk of a second heart attack.
- decreases risk of developing diabetes.
- helps regulate blood sugar and decreases risk of complications if you have diabetes.
- increases self-esteem.
- makes you feel happier.

Essential Play for Big Kids

Now, what do we mean when we talk about exercise? Our goal is to get you to move your body on a regular basis. It's as simple as that, but the issues involved are anything but.

First of all, by exercise we don't mean bodybuilding or an intensive training schedule. Most of us are not built for this physically or psychologically. Generally, we are not built to work out for three hours, seven days a week.

What we are built for is sport—fun and games, play, and competition. If you tell children to go outside and exercise, they are likely to just sit there and look at you. If you say "Go out and play," they go tearing around like crazy—they run, they jump, and they burn a lot of calories. If you put kids in a gym class and tell them to run, they hate it. But if you give them a soccer ball and say play, they're happy. They're meant to play.

So guess what? Adults are just big kids. We want to play, too. If we didn't have to work and have other responsibilities, an appreciable part of our day would be devoted to play and sport. Unfortunately, for most of us, our daily routines do not allow for kickball in the morning, tennis after lunch, and swimming in late afternoon. If they did, there would be no need to work out on a treadmill or stationary bike in the basement or garage. So, given our busy schedules, our realistic exercise options come down to home workouts or joining a health club. An active lifestyle should include walking, hiking, biking, swimming, and sex, and is great for enhancing your mood and quality of life.

Our goal is to help patients initiate and maintain an exercise program that focuses on the basics. We begin by getting them to walk, as we are fundamentally built to walk (we mean *walk*, not stroll). If you walk about ten thousand steps, or roughly five miles every day, that's all the exercise you need. Unfortunately, the average person walks about fifteen hundred steps, or half a mile—not even close to enough. This means you must take the time to *really* exercise.

Getting people to take those first steps is not always easy. As we said earlier, and it bears repeating, there are numerous excuses why people don't begin an exercise regimen: "I don't have time," "My hip, knee, foot, arm, head, etc. hurts," "I hate fitness clubs," "I don't want to do it alone," and "I just don't like it" to name a few. And there are others that are personal and would be considered embarrassing if disclosed, such as: "I hate to sweat," "I'm ashamed of my body odor," "I don't want anybody looking at me," "I will pass gas," "I may fall," and "I will fail at the attempt."

Whatever the reason for resistance or outright refusal to exercise, patience, encouragement, and unconditional support are critical to helping someone overcome their individual obstacle to do it. Two patients, Fred and Doreen, provide examples of what we mean.

Fred and Doreen

Fred suffered his first serious heart attack two days after his fifty-sixth birthday. He was treated with three stents and given numerous medications. He had steadily gained over seventy-five pounds since high school and weighed 245 pounds. He had high blood pressure and high cholesterol, both of which were difficult to control. The last time he exercised regularly was as a member of the swim team his sophomore year of high school. He now works as an engineer for a large pharmaceutical company. Even before his heart attack, he knew he was way overweight, out of shape, and had an unhealthy diet.

Every patient in our practice receives a cardiac psychological evaluation. As a result of his, Fred started regular therapy sessions that focused, in turn, on diet, exercise, and stress. After the first few therapy sessions, Fred became comfortable enough to talk about a prank pulled on him by his swim teammates that left him shaken up. He was made the victim of an end-of-the-year tradition where his swimsuit was removed in front of the entire girls' swim team and he was locked and left naked in the pool area. He was so traumatized that he did not return to the team the following year, giving some excuse for his quitting. From then on, he completely avoided swimming and anything to do with exercising.

He realizes today that his story may sound silly and embarrassing, but as he got older his nonexercising became easier. He admitted that he never before told the "depantsing" incident to anyone. Once he revealed his story, his shame and anxiety decreased and he gradually felt amenable to exercising and was willing to start a daily walking regimen.

Doreen's story has a similar ring. She was diagnosed with coronary heart disease at age sixty-seven. She, like Fred, had gained weight steadily over the years and currently tips the scale at 225 pounds at a height of five feet two inches. She has arthritis in her knees and ankles, resulting in swelling and pain. She has avoided exercise for two reasons. She says her legs hurt, and the more she stays on her feet, the more the pain increases. She also sweats profusely and is so embarrassed by this she refuses to be in public if there is any risk of sweating.

Efforts to help Doreen start exercising had to address these two issues. First, working with her internist, a new pain-management program was developed and implemented that lessened her arthritic pain and swelling. The medications enabled her to initiate a walking regimen that improved her flexibility, sleep, and mood. Second, she bought a used treadmill so she could walk at home and eliminate the embarrassment of sweating in public. She got on track.

What Is the Best Type of Exercise for You?

Like Fred and Doreen, many people have physical or psychological obstacles to exercising that must be identified and overcome in order to begin. After you accept the necessity of exercise, whether reluctantly or enthusiastically, you have to consider what the best type of exercise is for you.

The answer to this question is simple: The one you are willing to do. If you decide for yourself what you want to do, there's a better chance of your making a commitment to regular exercise. If, on the other hand, you are told to join a fitness club and exercise five days a week for thirty minutes, it won't happen if it's not your choice to do so. Often, what you are willing to do in terms of exercise, initially, is nowhere near what you need to do to improve your heart and overall health, but just starting to exercise is a huge accomplishment, and eventually your regimen will be better organized and more rigorous.

The Best Way to Get Started

Many people who begin an exercise program underestimate the physical and psychological importance of starting slowly. They're motivated and eager and go all out the first few days. Unfortunately, the result of this is too often burnout, or injury. And then it's all over. You never recommit. In order to avoid this, you must start slowly, a process that can take months before you are exercising at an optimal and safe level.

When Is the Right Time to Exercise?

Most of our lives are not set up to provide a specific, consistant opportunity for exercising. The good old days of recess and playtime are long gone. Now you have to carve out exercise time from your full schedule. Whether you work full-time, part-time, or stay at home, finding time to exercise is challenging but critical. For most people, there are only three times during the day to exercise: morning, midday, and after work.

For many, the right time is first thing in the morning, before breakfast. A workout becomes part of the morning routine: wake up, use the bathroom, then exercise. For others, the idea of getting up early and losing those last few precious minutes of sleep just to exercise is ridiculous.

Others prefer to exercise after work. Either you stop at the fitness club on your way home or you immediately exercise when you get home, before engaging your family. The longer you put it off, the likelihood of exercising goes down exponentially. When you go through the front door, don't give yourself permission to blow it off by saying you're too tired or too hungry, opening the mail, checking your e-mail and phone messages, playing with the kids, reading the newspaper, or discussing the day with your spouse. You know that once you find excuses to avoid exercising, it's all over for the day.

The third opportunity is to exercise at midday. Is this a realistic option for you? For some, using their lunch break to exercise—walking, typically—works out very well because it's like recess and happens every day at the same time. Midday exercise works out well for many people because it's time that's already carved out of their day and is free from work and family responsibility.

What Should the Frequency, Duration, and Intensity Be?

How many times a week should you exercise? How hard do you have to exercise to make it worthwhile? How long do you have to exercise each day?

The quick answer to these questions is: The more frequent, the more intense, the longer, the better.

First, let's dispel the thirty-minute myth. People somehow think that if you work out thirty minutes a day, three days a week, you've bought the golden ticket. Do this and you're completely protected. That may be true if you're ninety years old. The truth is, the more you exercise, the greater the benefit. Thirty minutes three times a week is better than nothing, but it doesn't get you much benefit for your heart.

The better answer is, you need to exercise at least five days a week, forty-five to sixty minutes each time, combining aerobic exercise (such as running, power walking, and cycling) and muscle-building exercises (lifting weights, sit-ups, push-ups, and pull-ups). This means forty-five to sixty minutes of pushing your body to exertion, where you feel your heart beating fast and you're sweating. The "talk test" can be used to describe the optimal intensity for exercise: When exercising you should be able to carry on a conversation, but with some degree of difficulty. If you can't talk, your intensity is too high; conversely, if you can talk easily, your intensity is too low.

Your target heart rate—a number calculated through gender and age—is meant to provide a guideline for how hard you should exercise. Some people assume that if you do not get to your target heart rate, you are not benefiting from your exercise. This is nonsense! If you are sweating and breathing hard, you are benefiting. Target heart rate is useful to help determine exercise levels; not reaching it, however, during an extensive routine does not mean failure. The eventual goal is moving your body forty-five to sixty minutes a day five days a week.

Where Should You Exercise?
Sometimes deciding where to exercise is as important as deciding to begin an exercise program. If your environment is not comfortable, you will either never start or not follow through with a meaningful regimen.

A comfortable environment can be in the privacy of your home. It could be walking an accustomed route in your neighborhood. It could be joining a health club where you feel comfortable. Or you could carve out a zone of comfort within a public environment. An example is one of our patients who has a body-image issue and finds it difficult to exercise publicly in a health club. She gets around this by removing her glasses (she can't see more than five feet without them), plugging in her music player, and disappearing within herself.

For other patients, choosing to join a club can be a definite plus. For them, exercising with other people is fun and creates a feeling of support. Others will shun what to them is an intimidating, self-conscious-making atmosphere and opt to exercise at home, using a treadmill, rower, elliptical trainer, or stationary bike. It doesn't matter which type of equipment you use—each has its pluses and minuses—as long as it's used regularly.

The problem is that within three to six months most people stop going to the club or working out at home regardless of the cost of the new equipment or the expensive monthly fees. Remember how motivated you were to drive to the club, or how excited you were to set up the TV and stereo system near the treadmill in order to alleviate the boredom of running for hours? Now, ninety days later you have an unused gym membership or a home exercise machine that's collecting dust. What's worse, when the bills come every month, you're reminded that you're not exercising.

The reasons why people stop exercising are the same reasons that they use for never starting (e.g., "I'm stressed," "I don't have time," "My foot hurts" . . .). You simply need to make exercising a priority regardless of your personal laundry list of excuses.

19

Getting Real about Your Weight and Diet

Most heart patients don't know they are eating all the wrong things at all the wrong times, and in all the wrong quantities. They often don't want to correct their behaviors or even want to know about it. However, they definitely do want to feel better. Here is an approach that will address the roots of the problem a little more honestly.

Know What You Eat

One of the most significant risk factors for heart disease and poor health is being overweight and eating a diet high in sugar, salt, fat, and calories. Unfortunately, this is the standard American diet. So, before we begin the tirade about all the things you need to do to eat heart-healthy, let's be realistic about the issue.

- By the end of the day, most people eat what they want, how much they want, and when they want, no matter what their doctor, book, magazine, or talk show tells them.
- Changing and improving your diet on a long-term basis is unlikely. Why? See the points mentioned above. You may make some small changes for about a week to a month or so, but long-term, permanent change is very difficult.
- Whether you need to lose five or a hundred pounds, if your diet consists of large portions of sugar-, salt-, and fat-laden foods, making significant and permanent changes will be close to impossible.
- Learning how to improve your diet and following through with what you've learned is about as pleasant as sitting in your car in traffic for

hours. Everybody telling you what, how, and when to eat is over-the-top annoying.

- If your goal is to lose a lot of weight, say sixty pounds, and keep it off permanently, you know this is challenging. You may lose it, but find it difficult to keep it off because sustaining weight loss requires skills, habits, behaviors, and a consciousness that most people have not learned. You have developed twenty to thirty years of unhealthy eating habits that don't get unlearned by dieting. You may have learned how to lose weight but not how to sustain the loss.

If you feel this is depressing or discouraging, you are reading this correctly. Trying to lose weight and keep it off is tough but it can be done.

In light of all this, what are you going to do when it is absolutely necessary to lose weight and significantly improve your diet?

First, you need to set realistic goals and realize that the key to success is not which diet you are on but modifying old habits. Second, you have to realize that any long-term improvement in your diet is good no matter how small or minor. And third, it's important to understand that improving your diet on a long-term basis is much more important than losing weight. The weight loss will come in time, but making positive dietary changes is far more critical.

Diet—The Knowledge Deficit

Cardiac patients can be described as falling into three groups regarding healthy diet and weight loss:

1. The first group thinks they have a clear understanding about healthy diet and weight loss, but in fact are completely clueless. They are difficult to deal with because they think what they're doing is OK, and that with just a few little changes they can lose a hundred pounds.

2. Patients in the second group admit to having some knowledge about a healthy diet and weight loss and are willing and open to learn about it. This group is easy to deal with.

3. The third group are the chronic fad dieters who continue to fool themselves and go from one diet to another, hoping the next one will work like magic. Deep down they know they need a lifestyle change, but they

create a history of diet cycling—weight loss followed by weight gain greater than the loss—that makes each new diet harder to do than the last one and long-term success more and more difficult.

Realistic Weight Loss and Health Tips

Several thousand diet books are published every year, each one promising you will lose weight fast and feel better by following the diet they recommend. What most of these books have in common is a description of the same critical guidelines for long-term success. Here are some specific tools that we believe will help you improve your diet, lose weight, and keep it off:

- Eat less food, that is to say, less than two thousand calories a day.
- Eat more often, five or six small meals a day, but not exceeding your recommended calories.
- Eat breakfast within the first forty-five minutes after awakening. Anything later than this is considered a snack, not breakfast. You cannot maintain weight loss without eating breakfast.
- Eat fresh foods. Lean meats, fruits, and vegetables should comprise 80 percent of your daily food intake (these foods are located on the outside aisles in your supermarket. The processed, high sugar, and high fat foods are in the inner aisles).
- Cut out sugar. Eat sweets only on rare occasions.
- Cut back on carbohydrates if you are eating too many of them. Reduce consumption of bread, bagels, pasta, muffins, crackers, pretzels, chips, cookies, and cakes.
- Eat much smaller portions at meals, especially in the evening.
- If you feel full, stop eating.
- Don't eat if you don't feel hungry.
- Break the habit of emotional eating and eating to relive stress.

Tips on Managing Emotional Eating

The fact is we are all emotional eaters, because we are all emotional people. Problems arise when we use food (primarily sweets and carbohydrates) to escape from or anesthetize our negative emotions and feelings such as anxiety, worry, sadness, guilt, anger, frustration, despair, agitation, irritability, annoyance, fatigue, and just plain stress. People who are prone to emotional eating usually start beginning mid-afternoon and continue through bedtime. Typically this is the time of the day when you become tired, irritable, hungry, and feel the effects of a stressful day. Emotional eating is truly about attempting to comfort yourself when you feel uncomfortable. Eating helps bring temporary relief, but once the food is gone, you often crave more, which perpetuates the cycle. These are the four keys to decreasing emotional eating:

1. *Get more sleep.* This improves mood and stress tolerance, and lowers stress hormones that decrease sugar cravings.
2. *Eat throughout the day.* Eat breakfast and focus on getting proteins throughout the day. Don't skip meals and become "Starvin' Marvin" at the end of the day. Curbing your hunger diminishes crankiness and stress, which also decreases sugar cravings.
3. *Learn to recognize when you are stressed, irritable, or anxious,* and choose a healthy food first to take the edge off before making the sugar choice.
4. *Exercise in the afternoon.* Exercising after three p.m. helps to decrease stress, manage sugar cravings, and improves overall mood.

If you are among the lucky few who can modify your behavior on your own and live according to these very healthy guidelines without help, then you are done. Most people, however, can't do this by themselves. It takes a great deal of will, focus, and understanding to modify all your ingrained behaviors and habits to reach a successful long-term outcome. For you, perhaps the only way to break the dieting cycle and follow the guidelines listed above is to get professional and expert support from a cardiac psychologist. (Note: Dieticians and personal trainers are also positive resources who can help you make dietary and health changes, but addressing the behavioral, psychological, and emotional components of eating is best addressed by a cardiac psychologist.) This will lead to a customized approach that will consider your individual habits, emotions, work, and family life.

Understanding Dieting

The lure of the fad diet is the weight-loss chase. It's fun and it's exciting, and as you lose weight you feel like a winner. The problem is that most people can only maintain any extreme diet for ninety days and a weight loss of fifteen to twenty pounds before their motivation falls off. As you stop losing weight, you get discouraged, a feeling of failure sets in, and before you know it, you've returned to your old eating habits. You gain back the weight you lost and even more, so, excited and motivated to repeat the process all over again, you start a new fad diet.

There are three main reasons for this pattern. First, the methods required to lose the first fifteen to twenty pounds are not the same methods needed to lose an additional amount. Metabolism changes, so exercise levels need to be increased, and adjustments to the diet are often necessary to continue weight loss. Most people don't have the knowledge or patience to make these adjustments, particularly when it requires additional effort over and beyond what the first three months demanded. Second, motivation is inherently short-term. Nobody can remain indefinitely and highly motivated. Thus, the correlation between continual weight loss and motivation; both appear to last about three months. Once motivation wanes or weight loss stops, the commitment to being on a diet ends. When the diet ends, people go back to their familiar habits, because people always return to what they know. The body often responds by gaining more weight above the prediet weight because the body is preparing itself for starvation when you eventually begin your new fad-diet all over again.

The Sustaining Phase

The diet books have it all wrong. You don't start with the sexy chase; you start with the sustaining phase, you continue the phase, and you never stop the phase. It is truly the most important part of any diet, but what is the sustaining phase? It means if a patient comes in weighing 260 pounds and wants to weigh 210, he or she is put on a diet for a 210-pound person—a diet calorically and nutritionally calculated to keep a 210-pound person at that weight. Eventually he or she will lose the weight to reach 210 pounds and sustain it (with cardiovascular and muscle-building exercising). It could take years. It's not a quick process and is not meant to be. Undoing years of bad eating habits and unraveling your psychological and emotional issues takes time, but it is doable.

Heart-Healthy Diet Overview

If you want to lose weight and improve your health, forget the fads and pills and learn to consistently eat as if you have already reached your goal weight and will continue to sustain it. You will be a winner; you will lose weight and continue to do so by making minor modifications in caloric intake and exercising. Here are some tips, questions, and answers that will point you in the right direction to a heart-healthy diet.

1. *What is a low-salt diet?* Stop cooking with salt. Stop salting your food. Stop eating salty snack food such as chips, peanuts, and pretzels. Stop eating fast food—it's loaded with salt. Stay away from salty canned soups and other processed non-fresh foods. These comprise 95 percent of your salt problems.

2. *What is a low-cholesterol diet?* Dramatically cut back high-fat and high-sugar foods such as chips, regular soda, fast food, pizza, fried food, candy, ice cream, and desserts. Red meat and eggs in moderation are fine.

3. *What meats are OK?* Fish and chicken are best, as well as lean beef and pork, again, in moderation.

4. *What is a healthy quantity of food?* For starters, keep a food log—write down everything you eat and drink with accuracy and specificity every day for one month. Amazingly, most people have no idea what they're eating and in what quantity they are eating it. Keeping a food log is a necessary first step for change. Often we find that a patient who is on a low-salt diet for high blood pressure will eat something

 Two Easy Ways to Calculate Calories

There are many ways to calculate calories, but these two are the easiest:

1. Go to the Web site sparkpeople.com. It is free and full of wonderful, helpful dietary tips. Input your daily food intake and the site automatically calculates your calorie intake. It also provides measurements of daily proteins, fats, and carbohydrates.

2. Take five standard cereal bowls and fill them up with food: meat, bread, fruit, veggies, and dairy. Once you've filled all five bowls, you have approximately eighteen hundred calories of food. This method helps to standardize portion sizes and helps to visualize a reasonable daily amount of food. If you are eating more than five "bowls" of food, you are most likely eating more than two thousand calories.

like a high-salt bison burger three times a week. Or a patient with a cholesterol problem will eat an entire box of doughnuts. Or a diabetic will drink a six-pack of soda each day and can't understand why his blood sugar is off the charts. A food log helps you identify what you're doing wrong and begins to influence how you eat.

5. *What is "portion distortion"?* What seems normal to you is probably too much. Begin by cutting portions in half and don't ask for seconds.

6. *Cut back on mindless snacking.* Snack foods are usually high in salt.

7. *Generally, eat less than two thousand calories a day* and you're moving in the right direction.

20

Smoking—It's All about Fear

The tobacco, medical, and cancer industries all tell you that quitting smoking is the most difficult thing you will ever do in your entire life. If you believe this, you have fallen victim to a con. In fact, becoming a nonsmoker can be one of the easiest things you'll ever have to do.

The Most Dangerous Risk Factor

Let's be perfectly clear. If we say that smoking is a risk factor for heart disease, all this does is sugarcoat the issue. In truth, smoking is a destructive force that clogs up the arteries in your heart and in the rest of your body. Think of it in terms of your bathroom sink. The more hair and other stuff you wash down the sink, the quicker it will clog up. Smoking is like throwing toxic sludge into the arteries of your heart. When those arteries get clogged, you are on your way to heart attack, stroke, or death.

Every smoker knows someone who smoked a pack a day for over fifty years and lived into his or her seventies, eighties, or nineties. If you believe you are one of those lucky ones, then you should fly to Las Vegas today and put your life savings on black. But for the rest of humanity, every time you light up a cigarette you reduce your life span.

For those of you who would rather have quality over quantity, then smoke as much as you want and enjoy your shorter life, but let's discuss that quality. Here's what you have to look forward to in your quality life as a smoker:

- Open-heart surgery or angioplasty.
- Numerous medicines—and their side effects—to control heart disease.
- Possible amputation of your foot or a leg, because smoking affects blood vessels more in the legs than any other part of the body.

- Severe physical and mental limitations from a stroke.
- Breathing difficulties from asthma, emphysema, recurring pneumonia, chronic bronchitis, and smoker's cough.
- Carrying an oxygen tank with you everywhere you go.
- Lung cancer resulting in lung surgery and chemotherapy, throwing up, chronic pain, inability to walk, chronic fatigue.
- Smelling like an ashtray—that everyone can smell except for you, unfortunately.

For the heart disease patient who smokes, it is critical that you understand that smoking is a very significant cause of your disease. There are other risk factors for heart disease besides smoking—obesity, diabetes, high blood pressure, high cholesterol, and stress—but smoking is the most important one. If you have heart disease and have had open-heart surgery or angioplasty and still smoke, be assured you are coming back for more surgery, even death. It's important to improve the other risk factors, but smoking is crucial.

Smoking Disinformation

So, how are you going to quit smoking and become a permanent nonsmoker? You have been told by credible sources that becoming a nonsmoker is a hard, uphill battle that requires one or more different methods—taking Wellbutrin or Paxil, chewing nicotine gum, or undergoing hypnosis—and that you know so many people who have tried over and over to quit and have always failed. The stories and the advertising get into your head and you're convinced it's futile even to try.

As a matter of fact, *trying* to quit smoking is the hardest thing you'll ever do because trying to do something is nothing more than giving yourself permission to surrender. However, *quitting* and becoming a nonsmoker is easy. Smokers are slaves to their cigarettes; *trying* to quit is another form of slavery. Once you quit, you're free. You have been conned into believing that if you quit smoking you'll experience terrible reactions that may require you to be immediately hospitalized, that you may go through convulsions, tremors, seizures, have so much stress that your head will feel like it's exploding. That if you don't have a cigarette available and the option of lighting up is taken away from you, you'll be so stressed that you won't be able to function.

All of this may sound way over the edge, but we've heard it again and again. And none of it happens. The truth is that smoking itself is the cause of your stress. You may think it's your spouse, your boss, your job, your children, or your lack of money. You may have some problems in your life (who doesn't?), but it's really smoking that's the root of your problem. Smokers spend a good part of their day thinking about when they're going to smoke, where they're going to be able to smoke, with whom they're going to smoke, when they can buy more smokes, what they will feel if they run out of smokes, and then actually having a smoke that takes three to ten minutes. Thus, 30 to 50 percent of their day is occupied with smoking. Once you end the slavery and free yourself of smoking, you can deal with your life more effectively.

How to Quit

So how do people successfully quit smoking? First, you must understand there are three components to smoking: addiction, habit, and attachment. Smoking is addictive because of nicotine, which, believe it or not, is nowhere as addictive as alcohol or narcotics. (You may read that nicotine is the most addictive chemical in the world, even more so than heroin. Nicotine is addicting, but there is plenty of debate as to its addictive strength. By the way, millions of people have successfully quit smoking, so maybe that big, bad nicotine is beatable.) Smoking is also habitual. After many years, the habit is developed to the point where a smoker does not have a thought, feeling, or action that is not associated with having a smoke. If you smoke one pack a day, you are having a smoke on average every forty-five minutes. Clearly, smoking plays an integral part in the smoker's life. And smokers form relationships with their cigarettes. They're like a bad boyfriend or girlfriend. You know they're not good for you, but you can't let go. Every time you try to quit, they talk you into taking them back.

Thus, you can understand why it may be difficult to quit, but you must do it anyway. You must face and overcome the fear that you can't handle your life without a cigarette. Most smokers say, "I like smoking," "Smoking relaxes me," "I work better when I smoke," and "Smoking reduces my stress." Smokers are terrified at the thought of giving up the perceived benefits of smoking. However, if you ask a smoker if he would go back in time and never start smoking, his answer would be unanimously yes.

The tobacco industry has conned everybody into believing that you can't quit without help. They tell people over and over how hard it is to quit, which makes quitting even more scary. Some people use quit-smoking aids such as medication, hypnosis, lasers, and nicotine replacements, but these help only if you have first dealt with your fear of quitting. Most people who once smoked and are now successful nonsmokers will tell you that they quit cold turkey and never looked back. They dealt with their fear. Something you should be aware of is that it's the tobacco industry that makes nicotine replacement products because they want you to stay hooked.

Conquering your fear requires total commitment: Pick a date and a time and make a public announcement when you will stop smoking. Don't analyze. Don't strategize. Throw out all cigarettes, lighters, ashtrays, and all paraphernalia. You will be terrified because you can't imagine not having your cigarettes close by. Nonsmokers don't keep cigarettes around "just in case." Just in case of what? Just in case you freak out and jump out the window, or go into shock, or have a seizure? None of this ever happens. If you really don't want to quit, there is nothing that will help you. If you're "trying" to quit—meaning deep down you know you aren't going to let go forever—you will become more and more stressed, making it "too hard" to quit. Eventually you will give up and light up. But once you do stop smoking, you will never turn back. You will have succeeded.

As a nonsmoker, there will be times in your life when you get the urge to smoke. But if you have conquered your fear and are no longer a slave to smoking, you will never start again despite your periodic urges. You might know people who did restart. Why? Because they never dealt with their fear. They might say they used willpower, but you can have all the willpower in the world and you will not be a nonsmoker. Stopping smoking is not about willpower; it's about understanding the con of smoking and your fear.

If you're looking for the holy grail of how-to-quit-smoking books, look no further than Allen Carr's *The Easy Way to Stop Smoking*. When you are ready to truly be free, let the cigarettes go and never look back. Remember, trying to quit is hard—actually doing it is easy. Hey, how about right now?

21

Getting Back on Track

Every heart patient needs a cardiac rehabilitation program, even though often most doctors won't tell you that. This supervised educational program does four things: It builds your confidence, it monitors your new medicines, it teaches you how to safely exercise, and it helps you feel that you're not alone. When your cardiologist refers you to cardiac rehab, be happy that he or she knows what's best for you.

Cardiac Rehab

You're lying in your hospital bed after angioplasty or bypass surgery and in walks a guy in a white coat named George. After introducing himself, he says, "I am here to start phase one of your cardiac rehab." You look at him blankly and think, *What is cardiac rehab? What is phase one? How many phases are there? Who signed me up for this? And who in the hell is George anyhow?*

To answer all your questions (except for "Who is George?"), cardiac rehabilitation is a supervised education program designed for cardiac patients that begins in the hospital right after your procedure and has three phases. Phase one, which occurs in the hospital, serves as the introduction into the cardiac rehab program. It is purely an educational phase that lasts the duration of the patient's hospitalization. Phase two is a twelve-week, three-day-per-week outpatient program that usually begins weeks after you leave the hospital. And phase three is a long-term, supervised exercise program that lasts for the rest of your life.

Of the three phases, phase two is the most essential because it gives you the necessary tools to start your new life. During the one-hour sessions, you are guided through a variety exercises, supervised by a cardiac rehab team that includes doctors, nurses, and technicians. During the exercises, patients are hooked up to a heart monitor that is continuously reviewed during the session. The exercises include walking on a treadmill or using a stationary bike and some mild strength training and stretching. This often provides tremendous comfort and assurance that the patient will not drop dead or have another heart attack during a workout.

A critical part of phase two is meeting with a cardiac psychologist and a dietitian. This is crucial because if you don't begin to address the real causes of your heart disease, which boil down to lifestyle issues such as stress, diet, exercise, and smoking, then you are never going to get better.

Also included in phase two are educational classes covering numerous important topics such as medications, anatomy of the heart, stress management, and nutrition. These classes are helpful because patients are given easy-to-understand and useful information for the first time regarding their health and medical condition.

We hear a lot of reasons why patients don't want to undergo phase two. They resist because it interferes with their work and their personal life, they don't want to exercise in public, and in general they don't think they need it. Also, many patients are convinced they don't have heart disease: "I don't have heart disease," "I didn't have a heart attack," "I just had one stent," "I don't need to be with all those heart patients." We don't agree. Every heart patient needs cardiac rehab.

The Faces of Cardiac Rehab

Typically, cardiac patients can be categorized broadly into three groups. The first group knows they need to exercise and work on their weight, but have just never gotten around to it. Once they are diagnosed with heart disease, they see cardiac rehab as a method to jump-start an exercise program and improve their life. The second group of cardiac patients is somewhat more difficult to treat because they don't want to go to a cardiac rehab and don't think they need to. In many cases, they think they exercise enough and pay attention to their diet. Clearly, they are in denial. Whatever they were doing hasn't worked, and they need rehab to re-educate and get them on track. The third group of patients needs rehab, but they don't get it because their doctor doesn't refer them to cardiac rehab. This group of patients is the hardest to reach because if their doctor does not emphasize the importance of rehab, they won't buy into the program.

Why Should You Participate in Cardiac Rehab?

If you're a newly diagnosed heart disease patient, the experience of a heart attack, going through bypass surgery, or having angioplasty is terrifying. You are probably afraid to begin any activity at all. You don't know your limits, and these need to be redefined for you. Exercising in a cardiac rehab program provides the comfort, safety, and guidance you need to begin exercising.

There are a few other reasons to participate in cardiac rehab as well. Being part of the program helps you build confidence, adjust to new medicines, and learn to exercise, all while you are under medical supervision. But, just as important, you benefit from feeling that you are not alone.

When you are diagnosed with heart disease, you will be given multiple new medicines. The types and dosages of the medicines need to be individualized for you, and this takes time. The monitoring process in rehab helps you and your doctor adjust the medicines more effectively and quicker.

Cardiac rehab teaches you heart-healthy exercises and how to exercise safely with regard to intensity, duration, and choice of exercise.

Rehab is essentially a support group. It provides relationships, support, and sharing with other heart patients. Newly diagnosed heart patients often feel isolated, scared, overwhelmed, and stigmatized. The twelve weeks of cardiac rehab provide a safe environment for you to heal. Be proactive and ask your doctor about your local cardiac rehab program.

Cardiac Rehabilitation Programs

Cardiac rehabilitation programs are supported and organized by individual medical centers and health-care facilities throughout the United States. Your local hospital or cardiologist can direct you to the nearest and most comprehensive rehab program in your area.

22

Treating the Whole Person

Each of the eight cardiac patients described in Part I is different (see pages 19 to 28). Therefore, we treated each one differently, depending on his or her particular issue, whether it was related to medication, a smoking addiction, poor diet, lack of regular exercise, stress, or a combination of these challenges. As we've stated earlier, we can't treat all the issues at the same time—they must be treated in the right sequence for each patient. And most important, our patients have come to understand that if we care, they will care.

Treating What Needs to Be Treated

Our philosophy of treatment is simple; it has to be individualized. No two people are identical; therefore, no two treatment strategies should be alike. Treatment involves a customized plan to deal with the five major issues involved in heart disease: smoking, diet, exercise, stress, and medicines.

While every patient does not have to address all five major issues if one or more is not relevant, identifying each patient's unique set of problems is critical. Most important, we must determine and then treat the patient's issues in the right sequence. Although the five components are all interrelated, we cannot and do not treat them all at once. The plan is to address all of them in due time. Everybody enters a treatment plan depending on what is right for him or her, and we continue to customize it to fit the patient's needs.

Barry

Here is how we treated Barry, our first patient profiled in Part I. Barry's key issue was stress. This impacted his diet and exercise, meaning he ate too much, he was overweight, and never exercised, but there was no point in trying to improve these habits until we dealt with his stress.

Stress ruled this guy's life. It was why he worked eighty hours a week, drank eight cups of coffee a day, and why his personal life was a mess. Why was he stressed? Because he was convinced that it was his destiny to die early like his dad and there was nothing he felt he could do about it. He lived in perpetual fear. Barry's dad died young, when Barry was just twelve years old. So he had his own secret timeline that no one else was allowed to know. Barry had to get everything done before he reached the age he thought he would die.

What did we do for Barry? We helped him face his fear, which resulted in a shift in his thinking. We helped him believe he was not his father, that he was making his own choices, that his life was his own, and that he had much more control than his father ever had. His fear will never go away completely, but it is under his control and not controlling him. It lurks in the back of his mind, but it is not in the forefront of his daily life.

Once he understood why he was accelerating his life at such a fast pace, he was able to start slowing down and change his diet, exercise more, and improve his personal relationships. Barry simply had too many bad habits. He ate fast, he skipped meals, and compensated with fast food and sugar binges. He didn't exercise because he said he had no time. He was in the thirty-pound weight club, meaning he was about 220 but needed to weigh about 190. He actually carried his weight pretty well, but he still needed to lose thirty pounds.

We first eliminated Barry's sugar binges at night, when it wasn't unusual for him to eat an entire sleeve of Oreos. This alone took off seven pounds. He was eating so fast on the run that he did not taste or enjoy his food. We had him sit and eat slowly and learn to taste his food. Enjoying the dining experience while eating less resulted in another five-pound loss. He agreed to start exercising and realized that getting his workouts done early in the morning, before seven a.m., made him feel better than ever. Another seven-pound weight loss. Overall, Barry is much better because, for the first time in his life, he is working on his issues and not living in denial. He realizes he has to work on his health for as long as he lives, and that there is no quick fix that will pay off over the long term.

Barbara

Stress was also key for Barbara, but in a much different way than for Barry.

Barbara is the matriarch and boss of her family. When she got sick, she regarded it as an assault on her identity. She felt that the entire family structure, built around her children, their daily and school schedule, her husband, his job, and his health, would collapse if she wasn't there to control everything. In her mind, she felt she was the glue that held everything together.

The root of her stress was overwhelming feelings of guilt. She felt that if she did not take care of everything and everybody, she was a failure. Taking time for herself was out of the question. Because she was so focused on everybody else, she disregarded her own health.

Thus, treating Barbara's heart disease required that she understand and manage her guilt. Once she realized that taking care of herself, even if that meant taking some time away from her family, would make her a better person, mother, wife, and friend. Only then did she allow herself to start working on her diet and exercise.

Barbara is a five-feet-three-inches tall, 180-pound, fifty-seven-year-old woman who was overcaffeinated and loved to eat bread. Improving her diet so that it would be more heart healthy and help her lose weight was very challenging. Barbara felt her only pleasures were her coffee and her favorite breads, so there was no point, early in her treatment, in getting her to eliminate these pleasures. It simply wouldn't work. A better approach was to help her move around and burn calories. Diet would be addressed last.

But exercise was a problem. Barbara is a woman who never wanted to exercise. She does not like to exercise. Her generation is a non-exercising generation. And to complicate matters, she doesn't like to sweat, especially in public. When she starts sweating, she stops moving. Barbara reluctantly made a deal with us that she would "try exercising" for two months. She carved out time at the end of the day to go down to the basement and walk on the treadmill. Now she walks forty-five minutes a day five days a week. She has not stopped yet. Also, her exercising has actually decreased her appetite for carbohydrates such as her favorite breads. However, she does permit special "carb moments" once or twice per week.

Bill

Bill would never admit, even to his wife, how scared he is of everything. The more serious the situation, the more he would be sarcastic and tell jokes to hide his true feelings. Having a heart attack, being told he has heart disease, having to rely on his wife, and being out of work were all overwhelming to him. Bill was not in a psychological place to start making lifestyle changes. But he did smoke his last cigarette before the paramedics took him to the hospital. The best treatment plan for Bill was to not push for major lifestyle changes early on, after he came home. It was important to help him get some normalcy and control back in his life first, by resuming driving, going back to work, and feeling independent.

Having a heart attack and going through surgery got Bill's attention, but it didn't last. Within three weeks, he began phase two, cardiac rehab. He did not want to because he believed he did not have enough time and that he could start exercising and dieting on his own. He was fighting change. Bill is a fifty-one-year-old man who is very comfortable with himself and his lifestyle. But it was primarily his lifestyle that caused his heart disease. He had not exercised since high school, he never cared about his diet, and smoking was part of his social fabric. Getting Bill to change was like breaking a wild horse. He had to accept that certain changes, which he believed were not to his liking, were inevitable. Once he reluctantly agreed to go to rehab, everything began to fall into place.

For the first time in thirty years Bill was moving his body on a regular basis. He cut out all fast food, which had immediate positive results. Without the excess salt, fat, and calories, the weight just peeled off. He felt better and more energetic than he had in many years. The combination of not smoking, eating better, and exercising made him feel like a teenager. Also, he realized that by carving out time for rehab he was able to shift that time to exercising when rehab ended.

Another key treatment point was identifying and treating his snoring and sleep apnea. Bill did not realize that his low energy and daytime sleepiness were due to sleep apnea, and that he used coffee, food, and cigarettes to keep him awake. Improving his sleep by helping him get an appointment with a sleep doctor (a pulmonologist who specializes in sleep medicine), who treated his apnea with a CPAP (continuous positive airway pressure) machine, really helped the whole process.

Rita

Rita got stuck in bad habits at the age of nineteen and kept on going—smoking, a fast-food diet, no exercise. The immediacy of life's pleasures and conveniences completely outweighed the long-term negative consequences. Forty years of neglecting her health resulted in arthritis, diabetes, chronic obstructive pulmonary disease (COPD), esophageal reflux (heartburn), lots of leg swelling, and finally a triple bypass.

Rita is used to not feeling good, but with swollen, aching feet and difficulty breathing she is more miserable than ever. To try to convince her that eliminating her main pleasures—cigarettes, coffee, and potato chips—would make her feel better would be a great waste of time, but this is the direction that had to be eventually taken. The key was a short-term/long-term approach. In the short-term, by markedly reducing the swelling in her feet, improving her breathing with medicines, and cutting back on salty foods, she felt better. For the first time she began thinking about making lifestyle changes. However, it was overwhelming for her to figure out what to do by herself, how to go about changing her diet, exercising, quitting smoking, and reducing her stress.

Working with a cardiac psychologist was her answer. A customized treatment plan was developed and implemented. Forty years of bad habits weren't going away quickly, but the guidance, support, and one-on-one attention proved to be the "medicine" she needed.

So what happened? The first issue to be addressed was smoking. Rita smoked for fifty years, since she was thirteen. She never tried to quit and never wanted to link her smoking with her lung disease and diabetes, and now her heart disease. Rita explained that smoking reduced her stress and helped her digest her food. She actually believed that smoking helped her breathe better and was therefore reluctant to quit.

She was willing to take a medication called Wellbutrin (Zyban), which reduced her stress, improved her mood and digestion, and reduced the withdrawal symptoms when she tried to quit smoking. The less she smoked, the easier she breathed, her legs hurt less, and she felt better. In addition, cardiac rehab helped her stop smoking because it bothered her that she had more difficulty exercising than other women her age. At first, she couldn't breathe while walking on the treadmill. But she realized that the less she smoked the better she breathed. She quit smoking altogether six weeks after starting rehab.

Rita was a clear-cut case of the benefits of getting rid of the junk food. Between the snack foods, fast foods, and regular soda drinks, she put away over four thousand calories a day (the average person needs less than two thousand calories). Also, her blood sugars were consistently over 160, which is way too high. Keeping a daily food record enabled her for the first time to see what she was eating. This significantly reduced her intake. She lost twenty pounds in six months and kept it off.

Rita remained invested in her care because every step she took made her feel better. She did not care about changes for future gain; she needed relief now. When she got relief, she bought into treatment more and more. Rita still has arthritis, her feet swell a little at the end of the day, and she still is overweight, but her life has improved.

Walt

The only reason Walt came to see a cardiologist is because he had bypass surgery and was told, when he left the hospital, to see one in a few weeks. So he did. He did not go intending to make significant lifestyle changes such as improving his diet, exercising, or managing his stress. Many patients after surgery or heart attacks are very motivated to do so. Not Walt. Walt was not interested in talking about his heart. He had just had major heart surgery, but all he could talk about was his back pain. When the topic of exercise was discussed, or weight gain, or sleep problems in reference to his heart disease, Walt wasn't concerned. His concern was his back. He said he could not exercise because his back hurt. He gained weight not because of poor diet but because he could barely get out of bed without feeling major back pain. And he could not sleep because his back hurt.

In addition to his back pain, depression was another issue for Walt. He just assumed it was normal to feel down and lethargic as a result of taking all his medicines. It never occurred to him that unresolved feelings of grief after losing his forty-two-year-old son in a motorcycle accident two years ago were a big part of the problem.

The only way to successfully treat Walt's heart disease was to successfully treat his back pain and depression first. He was open to treatment because we treated his back pain first, about which he was most concerned. We sent him to a doctor who specializes in back and chronic pain, treatment he had never had before. In addition, he had weekly cardiac psychology sessions that worked on his depressive issues. Only after he began feeling physically and mentally better was he able to participate in cardiac rehabilitation and start addressing his heart issues—diet, exercise, and sleep.

Alex

Alex had a bunch of things going against him. He had "bad genes" (serious heart disease in his family), he had given up on exercise when he was eighteen years old, and he ate an extremely high-fat and high-calorie diet. Putting these factors all together, he was destined for trouble. The good news was that any small and consistent positive lifestyle changes would lead to significant improvement.

Nevertheless, he had five stents in five years and still did not get it. Alex didn't exercise or improve his diet, and he resisted taking his medicines. It wasn't until his chest was cut in half during bypass surgery when he finally paid attention. For many heart patients like Alex, part of the problem is that stenting is too quick and easy. They come to the hospital, they go home the next day, and go back to their old lifestyle the following day. While a stent is a very successful treatment for chest pain, it doesn't treat the underlying problem of cardiac arterial disease, which is a progressive and chronic problem.

After his bypass, Alex was a very motivated patient. Also, the recent birth of his twin sons made him even more committed to getting better. He bought into a program of exercise, diet, stress management, and full compliance with taking his medicines. He never thought he had time to exercise, but now he realized that carving out time in his day for cardiac rehab was not as difficult as he thought it would be. In fact, exercising in the morning improved his mood, digestion, sleep, and energy levels.

He was up for making all the necessary lifestyle changes, but his diet proved to be the biggest stumbling block. His wife cooked to keep him plump. The key wasn't to send Alex to a dietician but to send his wife to one. She needed to understand and learn a heart-healthy way of cooking. As soon as she did, Alex became healthier—he was eating better and exercising. Unfortunately, it all fell apart three years later when he lost his job. At that point, he stopped exercising, lost some self-esteem, and he and his wife fell back into great tasting (that is, high fat and high salt) comfort foods. Over time and with much positive reinforcement, Alex slowly got back on track. His work situation proved to be very challenging as he was frequently laid off and each time he would give up on himself all over again. Cardiac psychology has helped in many areas, but he remains a work in progress.

Kevin

Kevin did not come into the office complaining of chronic pain, major stress, or depression. He came in because his primary-care doctor could not get his blood pressure under control. Kevin was on five different blood pressure medications and still his blood pressure averaged 170/95.

From a purely medical standpoint, this did not make sense. He was on more than enough medicines, but they weren't working. As part of the normal clinical routine, he saw a cardiac psychologist. Within a few sessions, it became clear that his main problems were chronic pain, stress, sleep deprivation, and depression, all of which were driving up his blood pressure. Kevin did not need another blood pressure medicine; he needed pain relief, more sleep, and an anti-depressant to deal with all of his problems, which were interrelated.

For the first time, therapy gave him the opportunity to discuss, work through, and solve his work and family issues as well as stress. The antidepressant helped his mood and decreased his pain levels, which resulted in improved sleep. He no longer needed twenty highly caffeinated cups of coffee to get through the day (reducing caffeine lowers blood pressure). Within three months, Kevin's blood pressure was under control with only two medicines.

Christie

Christie was run down and used up. She was over-sugared, overcaffeinated, and overmedicated. She had symptoms that looked like heart disease but weren't. Her palpitations, fatigue, and heartburn were directly caused by severe stress, poor diet, and physical inactivity. It became apparent that her blood pressure was only elevated in her doctor's office (white-coat syndrome). Her blood pressure medicine actually made her blood pressure too low throughout the day, which contributed to her low energy. She was taking cholesterol medicine that caused her joints to ache, which gave her another reason not to exercise. Ironically, the medicine Christie was taking was unnecessary because her cholesterol could be managed more effectively by changing her diet and getting her started on an exercise regimen.

Not giving Christie a diagnosis of heart disease and eliminating her medicines was the easy part for her cardiologist. However, this was not what she wanted to hear. Christie went to a cardiologist with the expectation of being treated for heart disease and given a cure, rather than being told that stress was her problem and that she should see a psychologist!

White-Coat Syndrome

This is a phenomena in which a patient's blood pressure is elevated only in their doctor's office. It is caused by the anxiety of seeing the doctor (i.e., "the white coat"). Outside the doctor's office, the patient's blood pressure is normal. This makes treating the patient challenging as doctors make medical decisions based on the blood pressure reading in their office. This commonly leads to overmedicating patients, which can result in a patient's blood pressure being too low.

Christie reluctantly set up a single visit with a cardiac psychologist. She had no idea what to expect, but she came away liking the fact that she was given a whole hour to talk about her life. This led to a second appointment, and then a series of visits that proved extremely productive. Christie began to make small but important changes in her life routine. She was still busy as ever, but she realized large benefits from small changes. For example, she explained that her only pleasure was her daily six-pack of Pepsi. She did not eat regularly; she lived in a sugar-saturated snack-food world. When she began to eat three meals a day and cut back on soda (she agreed to limit consumption to one per day), she started to feel better. But helping her open up and talk about her fears and frustrations was really the long-term issue and key to her health.

Through therapy, Christie began to understand and battle her fear of failure and constant feelings of inadequacy. Over time, she was able to achieve a better balance for herself and her family. Her palpitations, fatigue, and heartburn drastically improved.

This is a small look into our clinical world. It is our hope that the reader will identify with some aspects of our patients and their treatment. Successfully treating heart disease is very complicated and as stated above must be customized.

Epilogue

This book has presented the necessary elements to understanding and treating heart disease. It has been written solely with our patients in mind. They have told us time and time again what works and what doesn't work in treating their hearts, bodies, and minds. We have been honored to help and treat such amazing and dynamic people in our practice. We hope that *The No Bull Book on Heart Disease* provides real, discernible tools to help others successfully navigate their own health and the health-care system. Because most people, including our patients, live involved and busy lives, we believe they need a heart book that has practical, straightforward information and tools that they can actually utilize.

Successfully preventing and treating heart disease is complicated and for optimal results should involve the combination of a cardiologist and cardiac psychologist.

Actually caring, listening, paying attention, taking the time, and providing the right medicines and individualized interventions enable the powers of healing to take hold and work. Treatment must be tailored and presented in a way that you can actually use. Your own healing powers are unlimited. We hope our book is the right "medicine" at the right time to either keep you moving in the right direction or turn you around so that you will be.

Glossary

adrenaline: A hormone released by your body in response to a variety of situations—most notably, stress, anxiety, and fear—and commonly known as the "fight-or-flight" hormone. It is the survival hormone designed to help you run or fight a saber-toothed tiger in your cave. When released, it temporarily increases heart rate, blood pressure, and physical strength, and makes you sweaty and slippery.

angina or **angina pectoris:** Chest pain or discomfort, which occurs when you develop a blockage in one or more of your coronary arteries.

angiogram (cardiac catheterization): A test performed in the hospital that takes a picture of the coronary arteries to determine if a blockage is present.

angioplasty: A procedure where a blocked (or partially blocked) coronary artery is opened up by inflating a specialized small balloon in the blocked area.

antiarrhythmics: Medicines that help to normalize a patient's heartbeat.

anticoagulation: The process by which your blood is thinned. Typically this is done with one of three drugs: aspirin, Coumadin (warfarin), or Plavix.

anticoagulants: Drugs used to thin the blood, including aspirin, Coumadin (warfarin), and Plavix.

apnea: *See* sleep apnea.

arrhythmia: A condition in which a patient's heart beats irregularly, too fast, or too slow.

atrial fibrillation (AFIB): A disturbance in your heart's rhythm, a short circuit in the wiring system that causes your heart to beat irregularly and rapidly.

atrium: One of the four chambers of the heart. Its function is to receive blood from the body and pump it into the ventricles. There are two atria, left and right.

blood pressure: A measurement of how hard your heart is pumping and how stiff or relaxed your arteries are. It is commonly assessed by placing a blood pressure cuff on your right or left arm.

bypass (coronary artery bypass grafting; CABG): During open-heart coronary bypass surgery, new blood vessels are placed around a patient's blocked arteries, thereby "bypassing" the blockages. Surgeons may bypass between one and seven blockages, most commonly between three and five. Also referred to as a *cabbage operation*.

CAD: *See* coronary artery disease.

cardiac catheterization: *See* angiogram.

cardiolite stress test: *See* nuclear stress test.

chemical nuclear stress test: A diagnostic test designed for people who can't exercise. A chemical is injected into your veins to increase the heart rate, mimicking the exercise phase of a standard stress test.

cholesterol: A naturally occurring substance in all cells of your body. It becomes problematic when it accumulates in the coronary arteries, contributing to the formation of blockages.

chronic obstructive pulmonary disease (COPD): A disease characterized by progressive lung destruction and dysfunction, which causes difficulty in breathing. It is commonly associated with long-term smoking.

congestive heart failure: A condition in which the heart is not pumping as strongly as it should.

continuous positive airway pressure (CPAP): One of the treatments for sleep apnea is using a CPAP machine. It blows humidified air through your nose while you're sleeping. This requires wearing a mask on your face, which is hooked up to the machine that looks a little like Darth Vader, but is generally well tolerated.

coronary arteries: The blood vessels that supply the heart with oxygen.

coronary artery bypass grafting (CABG): *See* bypass.

coronary artery disease (CAD): Everyone has three coronary arteries that supply blood to the heart. Coronary artery disease (CAD) refers to the presence of blockages in those arteries.

coronary catheter: A long thin tube with a diameter the size of a pencil point used to visualize coronary arteries.

coronary thrombosis: A process whereby a coronary artery becomes blocked with a blood clot.

cortisol: A chemical produced by the adrenal glands that is involved in the regulation of blood pressure, blood sugar levels, and suppression of our immune system. It is released when we are stressed.

Coumadin: *See* anticoagulants.

CPAP: *See* continuous positive airway pressure.

CPK isoenzymes test: A blood test used to determine if someone has had a heart attack.

defibrillator: An electronic device used to shock the heart out of potentially lethal arrhythmias. It can be an external device ("the paddles"), or it can be internally implanted like a pacemaker.

diabetes: A disease resulting from long-term exposure to high blood sugar levels. Type-1 diabetics have some degree of pancreatic insufficiency that requires them to take insulin. Type-2 diabetics require different classes of drugs to control their blood sugar. All diabetics are at greater risk of heart disease, kidney failure, and eye complications.

diastolic blood pressure: When measuring blood pressure, you are given a top and bottom number. The top number is called *systolic*. The bottom number is called *diastolic*. The systolic number represents the pressure when the heart is contracting. The diastolic number represents the pressure when the heart is relaxing. The systolic number is always higher than the diastolic.

distal circumflex artery: One of the three main coronary arteries. It commonly supplies blood to the back part of the heart.

echocardiogram/echocaridiography: A diagnostic test that uses ultrasound waves to give a very detailed picture of how well the heart is pumping and a great picture of the heart valves.

ejection fraction: A measurement of how well the left ventricular chamber of the heart is pumping. A normal ejection fraction is considered to be between 50 and 65 percent. Don't be alarmed if you score less than 100 percent.

electrical cardioversion: It is a less-than-one-second procedure that takes place in the hospital while you are sedated that shocks your heart with "paddles."

electrocardiogram (ECG, EKG): A simple diagnostic test in which electrodes are placed on your chest to tell how the heart is beating, as well as providing information about possible heart problems.

gastroenterologist: A doctor who specializes in diagnosing and treating problems of the digestive system from your mouth to your anus.

high blood pressure (hypertension, HTN): It means your blood pressure is higher than it should be for your demographic and disease profile. *See* blood pressure.

Holter monitor: An ambulatory monitoring device that measures all your heartbeats for twenty-four to forty-eight hours, which is used to evaluate patients for palpitations and arrhythmias.

hormones: Naturally occurring chemicals in your body almost all made from cholesterol that are involved in practically every bodily function.

HTN: *See* high blood pressure.

hypertension: *See* high blood pressure.

hypertrophic cardiomyopathy: A disease of the heart muscle characterized by severe thickening of the heart walls. This disease has been linked to sudden death in young athletes.

intubate: A tube connected to a breathing machine is placed down a patient's throat into their lung to help him or her breathe.

irritable bowel syndrome (IBS): A bowel disorder characterized by abdominal pain, diarrhea, and constipation.

isotope injection: A nondangerous chemical that is used to visualize blood flow in the heart arteries (zero harm, zero risk).

myocardial infarction: Otherwise known as a heart attack. It occurs when a coronary is blocked and the heart muscle is damaged to some degree.

nitroglycerin: A drug used to help eliminate chest pain due to coronary artery disease. You can swallow it, or it can be dissolved underneath your tongue, placed as a time-released patch on your skin, or injected into a vein.

nuclear stress test: This test is similar to a standard stress test but provides a more detailed and precise diagnosis with the use of an additional isotope, either cardiolite or thallium (nondangerous chemicals that are used to visualize blood flow in the heart arteries).

open-heart bypass surgery (bypass surgery): A surgical procedure in which your breastbone (sternum) is cut in half and new blood vessels are placed around (i.e., bypassing) the original blocked arteries, providing a new blood supply to the heart.

pacemaker: An implantable device used for the treatment of certain cardiac arrhythmias. Usually, it is surgically placed just below the collarbone.

Plavix: *See* anticoagulants.

pulmonary stenosis: A condition in which the pulmonary valve (right ventricle pumps blood through this valve on its way to the lungs) does not function normally. It remains stuck in a semi-closed position.

rapamycin: It is one of the medicines used to coat stents to further protect against restenosis (i.e., preventing the artery from clogging up at a later date).

sinus rhythm: A term to describe the normal beating of the heart.

sleep apnea: It refers to cessation of breathing during sleep that can last between twenty and forty seconds. Commonly it is associated with snoring, obesity, congestive heart failure, and daytime sleepiness.

standard stress test (stress test): A test used to assess cardiac function. Typically a person walks on a treadmill for roughly ten to twelve minutes. Every three minutes, the treadmill gets higher and faster. The test ends when you can't walk any further, have difficulty breathing, or complete the test by achieving a target heart rate predetermined by your age. The entire time that you're walking or running, you're hooked up to an EKG that's hooked up to a computer.

stent: *See* stenting.

stenting: After angioplasty, a very small metal scaffolding is inserted in the artery at the site of the blockage (i.e., it looks like and is about the same size as the spring at the end your pen). This helps keep the artery open over the long term. A stent is left in the artery permanently.

steroid: A subclass of hormone that is involved in regulation and control of much of your body's metabolism and immune system, including but limited to: blood pressure, metabolism, sexual functioning, stress, and muscle and bone functioning.

stress test: *See* standard stress test.

systolic blood pressure: When measuring blood pressure, you are given a top and bottom number. The top number is called *systolic* and bottom is called *diastolic.* The systolic number represents the pressure when the heart is contracting. The diastolic number represents the pressure when the heart is relaxing. The systolic number is always higher than the diastolic.

thallium stress test: *See* nuclear stress test.

troponin test: A blood test to determine if a person has had a heart attack. Done in conjunction with a CPK isoenzymes test.

type-A personality: Normal human traits exhibiting behavior patterns of impatience, high competitiveness, hostility and aggressiveness, and an incapacity to relax.

type-B personality: Normal human traits exhibiting behavior patterns that are relaxed and non-competitive.

type-C personality: Normal human traits exhibiting behavior patterns that are pleasant, avoid conflict, and suppress feelings.

type-D personality: Normal human traits exhibiting behavior patterns that are anxious, irritable, and socially inhibited.

ventricle: There are two ventricles of the heart: right and left. The right ventricle receives blood from the right atrium and pumps it to the lung. The left ventricle receives blood from the left atrium and pumps it to the body. Patients with congestive heart failure have a problem with the pumping function of the left ventricle.

warfarin: *See* anticoagulants.

Wellbutrin (bupropion, Zyban): An atypical antidepressant commonly used for the treatment of depression and smoking cessation.

Zyban: *See* Wellbutrin.

Resources

Books

Bernstein, Richard. *Dr. Bernstein's Diabetes Solution: The Complete Guide to Achieving Normal Blood Sugars* (Boston: Little Brown and Company, 2003).

Carr, Allen. *The Easy Way to Stop Smoking* (New York: Sterling Publishing Co., 2005).

Koenig, Karen R. *The Rules of "Normal" Eating: A Commonsense Approach for Dieters, Overeaters, Undereaters, Emotional Eaters, and Everyone in Between!* (Carlsbad, CA: Gurze Books, 2005).

Rimmerman, Curtis M. *Heart Attack: A Cleveland Clinic Guide.* (Cleveland, OH: Cleveland Clinic Press, 2006).

Tolle, Eckhart. *A New Earth: Awakening to Your Life's Purpose* (New York: Penguin, 2005).

Tolle, Eckhart. *The Power of Now: A Guide to Spiritual Enlightenment* (Novato, CA: New World Library, 1999).

Williams, Redford B., and Virginia P. Williams. *Anger Kills: Seventeen Strategies for Controlling the Hostility That Can Harm Your Health* (New York: Crown Books, 1993).

Web Sites

The Cleveland Clinic Heart Center
www.clevelandclinic.org/heartcenter

WebMD's "the heart.org"
www.theheart.org

American Heart Association
www.americanheart.org

The Heart Truth
www.nhlbi.nih.gov/health/hearttruth/index.htm

Medline Plus: Heart Disease in Women
www.nlm.nih.gov/medlineplus/heartdiseaseinwomen.html

Heart Center Online
yourtotalhealth.ivillage.com/heart-health

Other Sources

Cleveland Heart and Thoracic Institute, cardiology patients' appointment line, call 1-800-223-2273 X46697

Dr. Joel Okner, cardiologist, or Dr. Jeremy Clorfene, clinical psychologist: call 1-847-856-8400

And, of course, in a medical emergency, call 911.

Index